Molecular Pathology Library

Series Editor

Philip T. Cagle

More information about this series at
http://www.springer.com/series/7723

Victor G. Prieto

Editor

Precision Molecular Pathology of Dermatologic Diseases

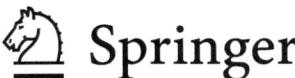 Springer

Editor
Victor G. Prieto
Department of Pathology
University of Texas, MD Anderson Cancer
Houston
Texas
USA

ISSN 1935-987X   ISSN 1935-9888 (electronic)
Molecular Pathology Library
ISBN 978-1-4939-2860-6   ISBN 978-1-4939-2861-3 (eBook)
DOI 10.1007/978-1-4939-2861-3

Library of Congress Control Number: 2015945659

Springer New York Heidelberg Dordrecht London

Printed on acid-free paper

Springer Science+Business Media LLC New York is part of Springer Science + Business Media (www.springer.com)

Contents

Contributors

Phyu P. Aung Section of Dermatopathology, Department of Pathology, The University of Texas MD Anderson Cancer Center, Houston, TX, USA

Francisco Bravo Departments of Pathology and Dermatology, Universidad Peruana Cayetano Heredia, Lima, Peru, Houston, USA

Su S. Chen Empire Genomics, LLC, Buffalo, NY, USA

Jonathan L. Curry Department of Pathology, Section of Dermatopathology, The University of Texas: MD Anderson Cancer Center, Houston, TX, USA

Department of Pathology, The University of Texas: MD Anderson Cancer Center, Houston, TX, USA

Doina Ivan Section of Dermatopathology, Department of Pathology, The University of Texas MD Anderson Cancer Center, Houston, TX, USA

Alexander J. Lazar Department of Pathology, The University of Texas: MD Anderson Cancer Center, Houston, TX, USA

Roberto N. Miranda Department of Hematopathology, The University of Texas: MD Anderson Cancer Center, Houston, TX, USA

Kudakwashe Mutyambizi Department of Pathology and Dermatology, University of Texas: MD Anderson Cancer Center, Houston, TX, USA

Victor G. Prieto Department of Pathology, Section of Dermatopathology, The University of Texas: MD Anderson Cancer Center, Houston, TX, USA

Department of Pathology, The University of Texas: MD Anderson Cancer Center, Houston, TX, USA

Michael T. Tetzlaff Department of Pathology, The University of Texas: MD Anderson Cancer Center, Houston, TX, USA

Department of Pathology, Section of Dermatopathology, The University of Texas: MD Anderson Cancer Center, Houston, TX, USA

Carlos A. Torres-Cabala Departments of Pathology and Dermatology, The University of Texas: MD Anderson Cancer Center, Houston, TX, USA

Wei-Lien Wang Department of Pathology and Dermatology, The University of Texas: MD Anderson Cancer Center, Houston, TX, USA

Chapter 1
Introduction

Victor G. Prieto

Although special techniques have been applied for more than a century to aid the diagnosis of pathology specimens, it is only within the past 10–20 years when the field of ancillary techniques has exploded to the current levels. From the beginning of histology and pathology, morphologists have used a wide range of special techniques such as silver stains to detect the presence of axons, colloidal iron stain to detect mucin deposits in the dermis, or Steiner stain to detect spirochetes. During the 1960 and 1970s, electron microscopy allowed examination of the subcellular structures to detect, among others, the capsids of viruses, organelles associated with a particular neoplasm (Birbeck granules in Langerhans cell histiocytosis), or alteration of the basement membrane area in the different subtypes of epidermolysis bullosa. Since the 1980s immunohistochemistry has become widely used to detect antigens, with applications to neoplastic (e.g., differentiation between Paget disease and melanoma), inflammatory (differentiation among the different subtypes of cutaneous immunobullous diseases), and infectious conditions (detection of spirochetes in cutaneous lesions of syphilis). In a sense, we can consider immunohistochemistry as an early "molecular" technique since it allows the detection of specific antigens (i.e., "molecules").

In the past 10–15 years, molecular techniques such as genomic sequencing have become much more available. From an original very expensive price and long-processing times, significant advances have much reduced their turnaround time and cost and thus have made them very attractive to diagnostic applications. The range of genetic or molecular tests that can be performed on skin specimens include polymerase chain reaction (PCR), fluorescence in situ hybridization (FISH), comparative genomic hybridization (CGH), gene arrays, routine cytogenetics, and mass spectrometry.

A very significant advance in the field of molecular techniques has been their progressive adaptation to formalin-fixed, paraffin embedded tissue specimens. As

V. G. Prieto (✉)
Department of Pathology, Section of Dermatopathology, The University of Texas: MD Anderson Cancer Center, 1515 Holcombe Blvd Unit 85, Houston, TX 77030, USA
e-mail: vprieto@mdanderson.org

© Springer Science+Business Media New York 2015

V. G. Prieto (ed.), *Precision Molecular Pathology of Dermatologic Diseases,*
Molecular Pathology Library 9, DOI 10.1007/978-1-4939-2861-3_1

it is well know, due to standard tissue processing (formalin fixation, successive heating periods, and embedding in paraffin), the genetic material is partially degraded so most tests were originally developed on fresh tissue or cell suspensions, thus limiting their practical use in dermatopathology. However, by developing successive modifications, many of these tests can now be utilized on standard, formalin-fixed, paraffin embedded tissue (the material most easily available in pathology departments).

As an example of the importance of these molecular techniques, genomic analysis has allowed to confirm that the old morphologic classification of lentigo maligna, superficial spreading, and acral-lentiginous melanoma correlates with a different genetic signature. Thus, melanomas arising in skin chronically exposed to the sun (i.e., lentigo maligna melanoma) have c-kit and NRAS mutations; melanomas arising in skin intermittently exposed to the sun (i.e., superficial spreading type) typically have BRAF mutations; and melanomas arising in the acral locations or mucosae (i.e., acral-lentiginous mucosal type) most commonly show c-kit mutations. Furthermore, this analysis has not only resulted in better knowledge of the pathogenesis of cutaneous melanoma but has also provided with identification of therapeutic targets in an area surely needed of new treatments.

In summary, this book reviews the most popular and useful techniques, in our opinion, for diagnosis, prognosis, and therapeutic purposes in the field of dermatopathology. Although almost any area of dermatopathology can benefit of the use of molecular techniques, they are currently preferentially used in some conditions, and thus this book devotes one chapter each to cutaneous hematolymphoid, mesenchymal, epithelial, infectious, melanocytic, and miscellaneous lesions. We are aware that it is certainly impossible to discuss all the possible applications of these techniques to the field of dermatopathology; however, we expect that this book will serve as a tool to familiarize the readers with these techniques and help them to add these tools to the diagnostic armamentarium in pathology.

Chapter 2
Hematolymphoid Proliferations of the Skin

Carlos A. Torres-Cabala, Jonathan L. Curry, Su S. Chen
and Roberto N. Miranda

Introduction

Molecular tests used by practicing pathologists are mostly performed on formalin-fixed, paraffin-embedded tissue specimens. Occasionally, when a more comprehensive molecular analysis is required, the use of fresh tissue or cell suspensions can overcome the limitations of testing on fixed tissue. The range of genetic or molecular tests that can be performed on skin specimens with lymphoid or hematopoietic disorders include, but are not limited to polymerase chain reaction (PCR), fluorescence in situ hybridization (FISH), proteomics, comparative genomic hybridization (CGH), gene arrays, and routine cytogenetics. In this review, we discuss the significance of the molecular testing most frequently used in the evaluation of clinical specimens involved by lymphoid or hematopoietic infiltrates.

Most of the molecular testing performed on cases of lymphoid infiltrates in the skin is done to identify clonality since it is generally thought that the presence of clonality supports a diagnosis of malignancy (i.e., lymphoma) and the lack of clonality excludes malignancy (i.e., reactive lymphoid hyperplasia). This approach is followed because it is considered that skin disorders with lymphoid infiltrates follow the paradigm of lymphoid disorders affecting lymph nodes, where evidence of clon-

C. A. Torres-Cabala (✉)
Departments of Pathology and Dermatology, The University of Texas: MD Anderson Cancer Center, 1515 Holcombe Blvd, Unit 85, Houston, TX 77030, USA
e-mail: ctcabala@mdanderson.org

J. L. Curry
Department of Pathology, Section of Dermatopathology, The University of Texas: MD Anderson Cancer Center, Houston, TX 77030, USA

S. S. Chen
Empire Genomics, LLC 700 Michigan Avenue, Suite 200 Buffalo, NY 14203, USA

R. N. Miranda
Department of Hematopathology, The University of Texas: MD Anderson Cancer Center, Houston, TX, USA

© Springer Science+Business Media New York 2015
V. G. Prieto (ed.), *Precision Molecular Pathology of Dermatologic Diseases*,
Molecular Pathology Library 9, DOI 10.1007/978-1-4939-2861-3_2

3

ality has usually been equated with malignancy. However, with further clinical specialization, increasing attention has been paid to lesions and tumors arising at extranodal sites, and differences related with specific anatomic sites have been identified, raising the concern that not all criteria applied to nodal lymphomas perfectly fit in extranodal sites. In dermatologic disorders in particular, whereas clinically typical malignant and benign lymphoid lesions exist and can be easily recognized by the clinician, there are many instances in which fully integration of clinical, pathological, and molecular findings is required to reach a definitive diagnosis. Apparent lack of concordance between these findings is a well-known, and probably not uncommon, phenomenon. Clonality may be detected in clinically indolent lesions (a "false positive," if following the paradigm of clonality being equivalent to malignancy). Conversely, clinically malignant lesions may lack evidence of clonality by molecular methods ("false negative"). Moreover, well-established pathological criteria useful for diagnosis of lymph node entities may not be applicable for their skin counterparts, such as the case of follicular lymphoma (FL), associated with t(14;18)(q32;q21) in approximately 85 % of the nodal cases (and usually positive for BCL2 by immunohistochemistry) but commonly negative for BCL2 and harboring the translocation in less than 30 % of primary cutaneous follicle centre lymphoma. The need for correlation of molecular findings with clinical and pathological characteristics of the lesions in dermatopathology cannot be overemphasized.

Molecular Tests Commonly Used in the Dermatopathology Practice

T-cell Receptor Gene Rearrangement Analysis

The T-cell receptor (TCR) is present within the CD3 complex that locates on the surface of T cells. Clonal rearrangement of the *TCR* gene is used to determine whether a T-cell lymphoid population is monoclonal or polyclonal [1]. The *TCR* is composed of alpha, beta, gamma, and delta chains. More than 90 % of the mature T lymphocytes harbor the alpha-beta TCR [2, 3]. It is important to remember that independently from what TCR (alpha-beta or gamma-delta) is expressed, rearrangement of the gamma gene is the most frequently detected in the T cells [4]. The *TCR* gene rearrangements occur in the following chronological order: delta—alpha—gamma—beta. Since the delta receptor locus is located within the alpha gene, the delta locus is deleted most of the times when the alpha gene is rearranged [5]. PCR-based methods—the most used in daily clinical practice—can detect rearrangements of the delta, gamma, and beta chains [6]. The gamma chain gene has less variation of sequences than the delta and beta genes, thus requiring fewer specific primers for the PCR amplification [7]. Moreover, *TCR* gamma gene rearrangements are found in both gamma-delta and alpha-beta T-cell lymphomas (in the latter, a rearranged gamma allele is retained although not expressed [6]), making the *TCR* gamma gene rearrangement detection the preferred test for detection of T-cell

Fig. 2.1 Analysis of rearrangements of the T-cell receptor (*TCR*) beta chain by polymerase chain reaction (*PCR*). The gene scan on the top shows amplification of segments as multiple small peaks and a large predominant peak. This pattern is consistent with a monoclonal population of T-lymphocytes. In the right context, this supports a neoplastic population of T lymphocytes. The *bottom* of the Figure shows a polyclonal pattern characterized by multiple small peaks, consistent with the presence of reactive, nonneoplastic T lymphocytes. *TCR* beta chain analysis is especially useful in the identification of a monoclonal peak in a polyclonal background

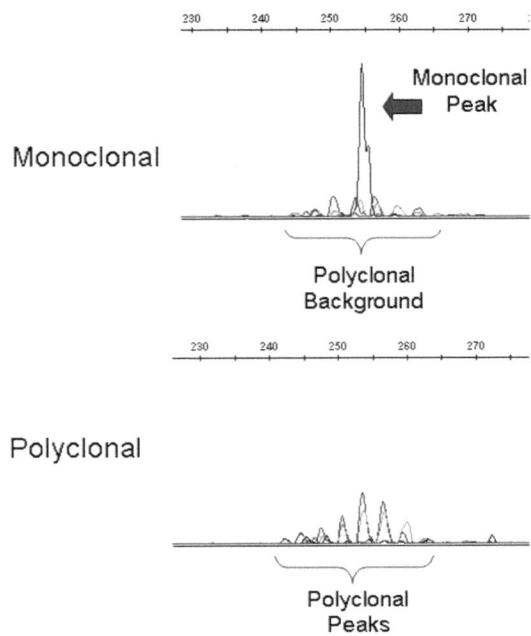

clonal populations in dermatopathology. Due to its greater combinational diversity, evaluation of *TCR* beta gene rearrangement seems to be particularly useful in the detection of a monoclonal population in a background of polyclonal reactive cells [8]. Rarely, cases of T-cell lymphomas may present rearrangements of the delta chain as the only evidence of clonality [9].

The PCR products are analyzed using high-resolution capillary electrophoresis. Polyclonal proliferations render multiple peaks (more than five) whereas clonal populations are characterized by one or two peaks whose height exceeds that of the polyclonal background by a ratio of 2:1 to 3:1 [10] (Figs. 2.1 and 2.2).

The sensitivity of PCR-based tests varies depending on the type of sample and technical issues. It is accepted that the minimum percentage of detectable clonal cells by this method is around 1 % [11] and that its overall sensitivity and specificity is around 70 and 97 % for mycosis fungoides (MF), respectively [12]. False negative results may be due to low numbers of malignant T-cells or absence of *TCR* gene rearrangement in the lymphoma cells [13]. False positivity (pseudoclonality) may result from amplification of *TCR* gene rearrangement present in a few T-cells composing a sparse, reactive lymphocytic infiltrate [14]. Duplicate analyses may distinguish reactive from neoplastic proliferations since the dominant peaks detected in reactive conditions vary within the same sample while true clonal peaks are usually reproducible [15].

In recent years, great value has been given to the demonstration of the presence of identical T-cell clones at different anatomical sites as a highly specific tool in discriminating between MF and inflammatory conditions [16], the so-called stable clonal pattern [14]. However, this pattern has also been reported in some

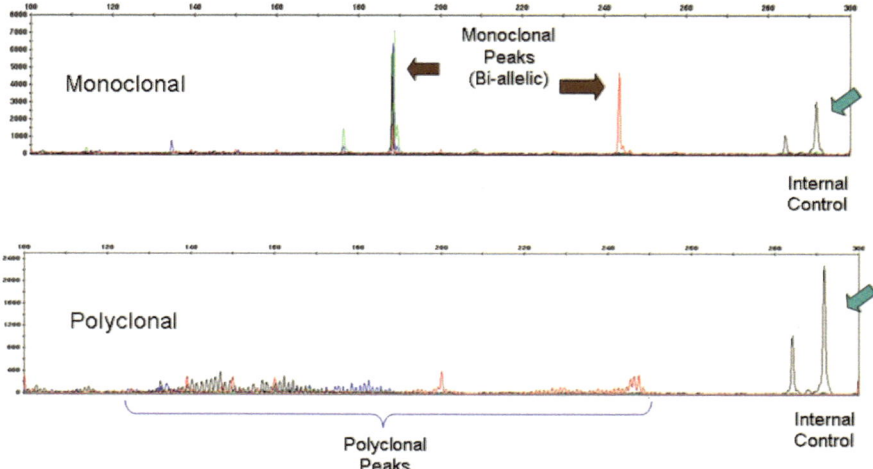

Fig. 2.2 Analysis of rearrangements of the T-cell receptor (*TCR*) gamma chain by polymerase chain reaction (*PCR*). In this case the scan on the top shows that the amplification of segments yielded multiple small peaks and two predominant peaks, consistent with a bi-allelic monoclonal population of T-lymphocytes. The *bottom* shows analysis of *TCR* gamma chain gene rearrangement in a different specimen. It reveals multiple small peaks, consistent with a polyclonal population of likely reactive, nonneoplastic T lymphocytes. As with the *TCR* beta chain gene rearrangement analysis, the correct interpretation of this result should be made in conjunction with clinical and pathological findings. The arrows indicate internal controls

inflammatory and "borderline" processes [17]. Conversely, genetically unstable subclones have been described in T-cell lymphomas [18] and clonal heterogeneity in MF lesions from distinct anatomical sites has been reported [19, 20]. The utility of comparing clones from different anatomical sizes for the diagnosis of T-cell lymphoma needs to be evaluated in the context of the clinical and histopathological findings.

Immunoglobulin Gene Rearrangement Analysis

The genes encoding immunoglobulins (Ig), the antigen receptors in B-cells, include the heavy-chain (*IGH*), kappa light chain, and lambda light chain genes. The *IGH* gene rearrangement starts with the combination of a diversity (D_H) segment with a joining (J_H) segment, which then is joined with a variable (V_H) segment to create a VDJ_H sequence. The kappa gene rearrangement then follows. Depending on the functionality of the rearranged kappa alleles, the lambda gene will be rearranged, usually after deletion of both kappa genes [21].

PCR-based methods for detection of *IGH* gene rearrangement utilize four sets of consensus primers designed to amplify three conserved framework regions within

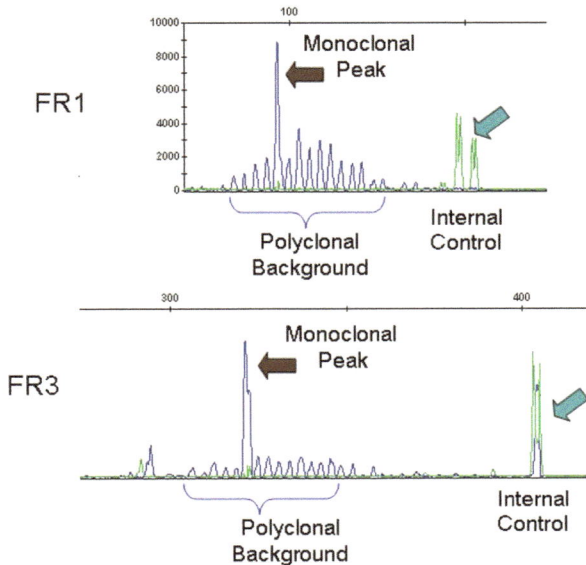

Fig. 2.3 Analysis of rearrangements of the immunoglobulin heavy chain (*IGH*) genes by polymerase chain reaction (*PCR*). Evidence of rearrangements of variable, diversity, and joining (*VDJ*) regions of IGH can be visualized by using pairs of primers at the V and J regions. Each lymphocyte in the analyzed specimen has a rearrangement that renders a segment that is amplified. In B-cell neoplastic processes, the presence of a prominent or distinct peak reflects that a significant number of cells in the specimen have the same size of amplified product. This finding constitutes a monoclonal peak and it usually correlates with a neoplastic expansion of B-cells. The use of three primers for the framework region (*FR*) of the V regions yields a higher chance of identifying a monoclonal population. The top of the figure shows the results of PCR amplification using FR1 and J region primers, while the bottom shows the amplification using FR3 and J region primers. Both analyses yielded the identification of a monoclonal peak amidst several smaller peaks, indicating that the neoplastic clone is admixed with reactive B lymphocytes. The size of the amplified segment is 98 base pairs on the top and is 320 base pairs on the bottom. Internal controls are used to confirm the size of segments and that amplification is taking place. The arrows indicate internal controls

V_H and one within J_H. From these, PCR amplification of framework region III in the V_H and the framework region in J_H segments is the most widely used test in clinical practice, due to the low molecular weight of the resulting amplicon and therefore the possibility of using formalin-fixed paraffin-embedded tissue as DNA source [22].

Same as for *TCR* gene rearrangement analysis, the peaks obtained by capillary electrophoresis are evaluated for the presence of a dominant population or populations (Figs. 2.3 and 2.4). The sensitivity of the method, although usually high, varies according to a number of factors such as the number of reactive B-cells present in the background and tissue fixation, and it can be as low as 47 % in formalin-fixed paraffin-embedded tissue [23]. The rate of false negative results seems to be espe-

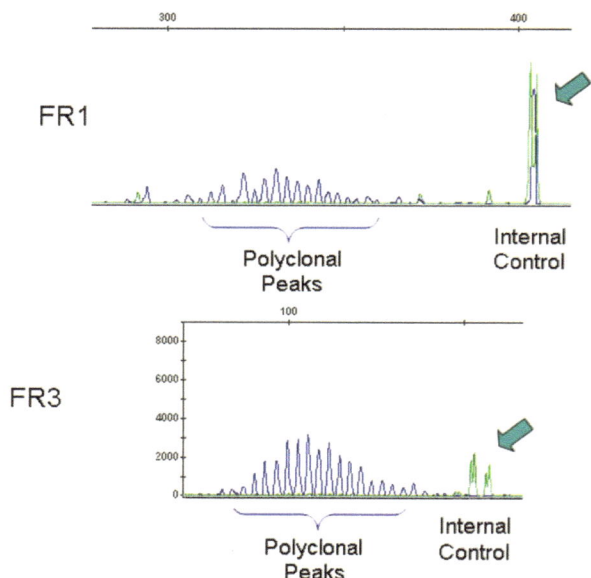

Fig. 2.4 Analysis of rearrangements of the immunoglobulin heavy chain (*IGH*) genes by polymerase chain reaction (*PCR*). In a reactive process, most lymphocytes render different size of amplified product and appear as multiple peaks, interpreted as polyclonal peaks/polyclonal background. In this case, the amplification of segments using FR1 and FR3 primers revealed a polyclonal pattern, consistent with a reactive, not neoplastic infiltrate. Similar results were obtained using FR2 primers. Correlation with clinical and pathological findings is still needed for an adequate interpretation of results of *IGH* gene rearrangement analysis. The arrows indicate internal controls.

cially high in cases of diffuse large B-cell lymphoma (DLBL) and follicular lymphoma, which have a high frequency of somatic mutations [24]. These mutations lead to sequences that are noncomplementary to the primer sequences. Such false-negative result is avoided by using multiple PCR target regions such as FR1, FR2, and FR3 segments of *IGH* gene. Another way to increase the sensitivity to detect clonal B-cell populations is by adding a test for immunoglobulin light chain (IGL) kappa or lambda gene rearrangement [25].

False positive results may be seen in cases in which the skin biopsy shows only sparse infiltrate and the PCR products amplified from the few B-cells appear as a distinct peak. Again, as for T-cell pseudoclonal cases, repeated testing may help in discriminating false clonality from true clonal B-cell expansion. Cases of cutaneous lymphoid hyperplasia have been demonstrated to be clonal for *IGH* gene rearrangement [26], and clonal *IGH* gene rearrangement has been reported in T-cell proliferations [27]. Other causes of false-positive results include immune disorders and infections showing a predominant B-cell population.

It is important to emphasize that the demonstration of monoclonal *IGH* or *TCR* gene rearrangement in a cutaneous lymphoid proliferation by itself does not make

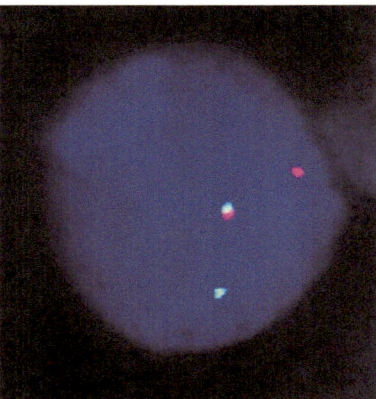

Fig. 2.5 Break-apart fluorescence in situ hybridization (*FISH*) analysis for identification of translocations involving *DUSP22-IRF4* gene locus. The picture shows a nucleus of a cutaneous anaplastic large cell lymphoma (*C-ALCL*) cell in which there is separation of *red* and *green* signals flanking the locus containing the *DUSP22* and *IRF4* genes, indicating a translocation involving this locus. This finding is most often seen in primary cutaneous ALCL, though it may be seen occasionally in systemic ALK-negative ALCL. (Courtesy of Dr. Andrew L. Feldman, Mayo Clinic, Rochester, MN, USA)

the diagnosis of lymphoma, and that both positive and negative results need to be interpreted in the appropriate clinical and histopathological context.

Detection of Chromosomal Translocations

From the several chromosomal translocations identified in hematolymphoid proliferations only a few are routinely investigated in the dermatopathology practice.

The t(14:18)(q32;q21) *IGH/BCL2* translocation can be analyzed by FISH and PCR. Fluorescence in situ hybridization (FISH), using appropriate probes, can detect almost all *BCL2* translocations [28]. This translocation occurs in more than 85% of cases of follicular lymphoma [29] but in only a small number of primary follicular lymphomas of the skin [30], and therefore its presence should suggest secondary involvement of the skin by systemic follicular lymphoma.

Translocations associated with extranodal marginal zone lymphoma rarely occur in the primary cutaneous tumors. The t(14:18)(q32;q21) *MALT1/IGH* has been identified in a subset of extranodal marginal zone lymphomas of the skin [31].

The t(2;5)(p23;q35)*ALK/NPM,* found in most of the cases of systemic anaplastic large cell lymphoma (ALCL) [32], has been rarely reported in primary cutaneous ALCL [33]. The demonstration of *ALK* gene rearrangements by FISH is thus very suggestive of secondary cutaneous involvement by systemic ALK+ ALCL [34]. A subset of primary cutaneous ALCL harbors (interferon regulatory factory-4) translocations; [35] FISH testing in this setting may be of potential diagnostic utility (Fig. 2.5) .

In situ Hybridization Studies

Demonstration of cytoplasmic immunoglobulin (Ig) light chain mRNA in plasma cells can be achieved by in situ hybridization (ISH) studies performed on formalin-fixed paraffin-embedded tissue sections [36]. Restricted Ig lambda or kappa light chains support a diagnosis of extranodal marginal zone lymphoma.

Epstein-Barr virus-encoded mRNA (EBER) ISH studies are important in a number of T-cell and B-cell lymphoproliferative disorders and lymphomas. Latent Epstein-Barr virus (EBV) infection can be revealed by ISH studies due to the large load of EBERs present in the nuclei of infected cells [37].

T-cell Lymphoid Proliferations of the Skin

Mycosis Fungoides

Mycosis fungoides (MF) is the most common cutaneous T-cell lymphoma. Clinical features are crucial for diagnosing this entity, especially on its early stages. The initial presentation is that of small scaly patches, usually on sun-protected areas such as the buttocks, lower abdomen, and thighs. In a minority of patients the patches disseminate and indurated raised plaques appear. The third stage is called tumor stage, which results in nodules that frequently ulcerate and may involve sun-exposed skin. Extracutaneous dissemination may be seen as the disease progresses. The histopathological findings on early, patch-stage mycosis fungoides are subtle and can be easily overlooked. The lymphocytic infiltrate is usually composed of small lymphocytes with minimal or no atypia, arranged around vessels within the papillary dermis and superficial plexus. Epidermotropism by lymphocytes, considered a strong sign for suspecting MF (especially in the absence of important spongiosis), may be very focal. As the lesion progresses, the lymphocytes start to display more obvious cytologic atypia. Plaques of MF usually exhibit cells with "cerebriform" nuclei and often show Pautrier's microabscesses. Dense infiltrates occupying the reticular dermis characterize tumor lesions. The lymphocytes in tumor stage MF may display an anaplastic morphology making the distinction between MF and ALK negative anaplastic large cell lymphoma (ALCL) impossible without clinical information. Many clinical and histopathological variants of MF have been described. Although scoring systems using clinical, histopathological, immunophenotypic, and molecular characteristics are in use [38], the diagnosis of early MF can still be cumbersome.

Staging of MF, mainly based on clinical and histopathological findings, correlates with prognosis [39]. Immunophenotyping is used as an adjunct for diagnosis. Most of the cases display a CD3+, CD4+, CD8− phenotype. Demonstration of loss of CD2, CD3, CD5, or CD7 may help in the diagnosis [11]. However, some controversy still exists about the exact role of immunohistochemistry in the diagnosis of early MF, since overlapping findings may be seen in inflammatory conditions [40] and the prognosis of early MF does not seem to be influenced by phenotype [41].

Molecular studies can be helpful in the diagnosis of MF, if taken in conjunction with clinical and histopathological findings. T-cell receptor (*TCR*) gene rearrangement studies are used to demonstrate T-cell clonality in MF [42]. Although Southern blot analysis is still considered the gold standard for determination of T-cell clonality, [43] PCR-based methods are routinely used for this purpose. Investigation of TCR-γ chain gene rearrangements is the most commonly used test in clinical laboratories, due to its high sensitivity [44, 45]. Evaluation of *TCR*-β gene rearrangements is being increasingly performed in clinical settings. It is expected that the assessment of both *TCR*-γ and *TCR*-β gene rearrangements will increase the sensitivity of T-cell clonality detection in MF [8].

When interpreting *TCR* gene rearrangement studies the dermatopathologist should be aware of a few caveats. Inflammatory conditions in which the lymphocytic infiltrates are scant not uncommonly yield oligoclonal or even monoclonal bands [3]. Duplicate analyses are needed to rule out the possibility of pseudoclonality in these cases [14]. On the other hand, the sensitivity of the PCR-based methods used for *TCR* gene rearrangement determination widely varies: it is not uncommon that patch MF lesions show oligoclonality [14]. Therefore, a negative or oligoclonal *TCR* gene rearrangement pattern does not rule out MF.

Sézary Syndrome

Sézary syndrome (SS) is characterized by erythroderma, lymphadenopathy, and the presence of the so-called Sézary cells in peripheral blood. Controversy still exists about the distinction between erythrodermic MF (a condition that may evolve through patch/plaque disease and has variable levels of blood involvement) and SS [46]. Some evidence suggests that these are two different processes and that they constitute malignancies of thymic memory T cells (SS) and skin resident effector memory T cells (MF) [47]. The prevailing view of SS as the leukemic counterpart of MF seems therefore not completely accurate. On clinical grounds, however, there is frequent overlapping between these two entities and a diagnosis of SS should be made under strict criteria, such as the demonstration of a T-cell clone in peripheral blood, peripheral blood lymphocytosis with a CD4+/CD8+ ratio greater than 10, and circulating Sézary cells greater than 1×10^9/L.

Histologically, the changes seen in SS may be indistinguishable from those seen in MF. However, lack of epidermotropism and low grade cytologic atypia are common in SS [48]. Most of the cases exhibit a CD3+, CD4+, CD8− phenotype.

Clonal *TCR* gene rearrangements are commonly demonstrated in peripheral blood of patients with SS [1]. These monoclonal *TCR* gene rearrangements can be identical to those detected in skin [49] and this finding has been used as evidence of multiple site involvement by the same malignant process. However, different clonal *TCR* gene rearrangements in peripheral blood and skin have been detected in a number of patients, suggesting clonal heterogeneity in some cases [14, 19].

Moreover, monoclonal T-cell populations in peripheral blood have been associated with autoimmune disorders [17], advanced age [50], and can be identified in association with other non cutaneous lymphomas and inflammatory skin conditions [1]. Patients with SS may be negative for T-cell clones in peripheral blood [51].

Primary Cutaneous CD30-Positive T-cell Lymphoproliferative Disorders

Primary cutaneous CD30-positive T-cell lymphoproliferative disorders (CD30+ TLPD) constitute the second most common cutaneous T-cell lymphoma/lymphoid proliferations. The WHO classification recognizes three types: primary cutaneous anaplastic large cell lymphoma (C-ALCL), lymphomatoid papulosis (LyP), and borderline lesions. It is recognized that these disorders represent a clinical and histological spectrum of entities going from LyP, a recurrent, benign diffuse eruption of papulonodular lesions that regress spontaneously, to C-ALCL, usually presenting as one or multiple localized ulcerated nodules they may in some cases regress [52]. Distinction should be made from systemic ALCL with secondary involvement of the skin and from other lymphomas showing CD30 expression, such as mycosis fungoides with large cell transformation [53].

LyP has been classified classically in three histological types [54]. Type A, that resembles Hodgkin lymphoma, i. e., shows aggregates of large Reed-Sternberg-like CD30-positive cells in a background of inflammatory cells; type B, or papular mycosis fungoides-like; and type C, or ALCL-like in which the large CD30-positive cells are arranged in sheets with minimal inflammatory background. Recently, a "type D" denomination has been proposed for CD8-positive lesions [55]. Cutaneous anaplastic large cell lymphoma (C-ALCL) reveals a dermal infiltrate composed of large anaplastic, pleomorphic cells, most of them expressing CD30.

The demonstration of clonal rearrangements of TCR in CD30+ TLPD has been variably reported [56, 57]. It is important to take in consideration that identical clones can be detected in different CD30+ TLPD lesions [58] as well as in LyP and concomitant lesions of mycosis fungoides [57]. When dealing with ALCL lesions, it is important to distinguish C-ALCL from involvement of skin by systemic ALCL. Cutaneous anaplastic large cell lymphoma (C-ALCL) cases usually lack t(2;5) and ALK expression by immunohistochemistry [59]. Translocations involving IRF4 detected in C-ALCL but not in systemic ALCL, have been reported as useful in this differential diagnosis [35].

Other Primary Cutaneous T-Cell and NK Lymphomas

This group encompasses rare lymphomas in which a diagnosis of MF has been excluded, clinically and histopathologically.

Primary cutaneous pleomorphic CD4-positive small/medium sized T-cell lymphoma is a provisional category in the 2008 WHO classification. There is controversy about whether this entity should be considered a true lymphoma or an atypical lymphoid proliferation of undetermined significance [60]. It presents as a single or multiple localized lesions on the upper trunk, neck, or face. The course is usually indolent although some aggressive cases have been reported [61]. Histologically, a dermal infiltrate composed of small to medium-sized T cells expressing CD4 admixed with numerous B cells, variable number of CD8-positive T cells, plasma cells, eosinophils, and histiocytes, is present. Expression of BCL6, PD-1, and CXCL13 has been reported in these cases and linked this lesion to a possible follicular T helper origin [62]. In a large series of cases, 60 % of cases were found to have a monoclonal rearrangement of the TCR gamma [60].

Primary cutaneous CD8-positive aggressive epidermotropic cytotoxic T-cell lymphoma (Berti's lymphoma) on the other hand, is characterized by multiple skin nodules that rapidly disseminate [63]. The prognosis is usually poor. On histological examination, the tumor cells—which can range from small to large—show marked epidermotropism and cytotoxic phenotype. Monoclonal *TCR* gene rearrangement has been reported in most of the few reported cases [64, 65].

Subcutaneous panniculitis-like T-cell lymphomas (SPTCL) include only cases with the alpha-beta phenotype [66]. Patients usually present with nodules or plaques on lower extremities with or without systemic symptoms. A common association with hemophagocytic syndrome was originally reported [67]. The skin biopsies show a lobular panniculitis pattern. Epidermal or marked dermal involvement is uncommon. The infiltrating cells are an admixture of small, medium, or large cells with variable numbers of histiocytes. Rimming of adipocyte spaces by lymphoma cells, erythrophagocytosis, fat necrosis, and karyorrhexis is variably seen. The atypical cells express CD3 and CD8 and are usually negative for CD4. Distinction of this entity from inflammatory conditions such as lupus erythematosus profundus, Weber-Christian disease, histiocytic cytophagic panniculitis, and reactive panniculitis to drugs or injections can be very challenging. Molecular analysis of *TCR* gene rearrangement helps in the differential diagnosis, since most of the cases of SPTCL are monoclonal [68].

Primary cutaneous gamma-delta T-cell lymphoma is an aggressive tumor that occurs in young adults and presents with multiple lesions, commonly on proximal lower extremities, and shows frequent mucosal involvement [69]. Three histologic patterns have been described: epidermotropic, dermal, and subcutaneous [70, 71]. These patterns may be observed within a single biopsy. Epidermotropism may be present. Rimming of adipocytes, similar to that seen in SPTCL, may be seen [70]. The tumor cells have a cytotoxic phenotype, with strong expression of granzyme B, TIA-1, and perforin. The T-cell phenotype of the tumor cells is confirmed by expression of CD3. The cells are usually double negative for CD4 and CD8, [72] although CD8 expression has been observed in some cases. CD56 is commonly positive. The tumor cells are negative for βF1 and positive for TCRγ and TCRδ by immunohistochemistry (the latter requires frozen tissue.) Most of the cases show monoclonal *TCR* gene rearrangement [71].

Cutaneous adult T-cell leukemia/lymphoma (ATLL) refers to skin-limited lesions without lymph node or peripheral blood involvement [73, 74]. ATLL is endemic in Japan, the Caribbean islands, South America, and regions of Central Africa. It is caused by the human T-cell leukemia virus type I (HTLV-1) [73]. Secondary cutaneous involvement is frequently seen in the systemic form. On histologic examination, ATLL cells in skin display a predominantly perivascular distribution and varying degrees of epidermotropism in a pattern sometimes indistinguishable from that seen in mycosis fungoides. The tumor cells are positive for CD3, CD4, and CD25 [75]. Monoclonal integration of HTLV-1 proviral DNA can be detected by Southern blot analysis in most cases of ATLL [76]. Interestingly, extraordinary integration patterns of HTLV-1 proviral DNA are associated with distinct clinical and pathological subtypes and prognosis [77].

Primary cutaneous extranodal NK/T-cell lymphoma, nasal type includes NK-cell lymphomas along with some cytotoxic T-cell lymphomas and lymphomas with indeterminate lineage (NK/T) [78]. These tumors, although rare in Western populations, are not uncommonly seen in Asian and Latin American countries [79–81]. Associated EBV infection is detected in almost all the cases [82, 83]. Patients are present with multiple ulcerated nodules with necrotic centers. The prognosis is poor [84]. Histologically, the lesions show a dense dermal infiltrate of variably sized cells with angiocentric distribution and necrosis [85]. Subcutaneous infiltration by the lymphoma cells, similar to that seen in SPTCL, can be seen. The tumor cells are usually positive for CD56, cytoplasmic CD3, and cytotoxic markers. It is important to demonstrate the presence of EBV, commonly by EBER ISH testing. T-cell receptor (*TCR*) gene rearrangement is not detected in the true NK-cell neoplasms; however, a subset of cases shows monoclonal *TCR* gene rearrangements [86, 87]. Assessment of the NK-cell killer immunoglobulin-like receptor (KIR) repertoire through reverse transcriptase PCR has been used to demonstrate monoclonality in these tumors [88].

Another EBV-associated lymphoid proliferation with distinct clinical presentation, regarded in the WHO/EORTC classification as a variant of the previous category, is the *hydroa vacciniforme-like cutaneous T-cell lymphoma (HVLL)* [89]. It usually affects children and young adults and occurs in regions of Latin America and Asia [90, 91]. Patients present with vesicles and papules on sun-exposed areas that leave scars clinically resemble hydroa vacciniforme. Hypersensitivity to mosquito bites is common. It seems that this disease is a part of the spectrum of EBV-related T-cell lymphoid proliferations of the skin that may include typical hydroa vacciniforme and aggressive lymphomas [92]. The proliferating cells in HVLL usually express CD3, CD2, CD8, and cytotoxic markers. T-cell receptor (*TCR*) gene rearrangement is detected in a variable proportion of cases [93, 94]. Detection of EBER-1 and *Bam*HI A rightward transcripts (BARTs) by real time PCR from skin crusts and scales of patients with EBV-associated cutaneous lesions has been reported as highly sensitive and specific [95].

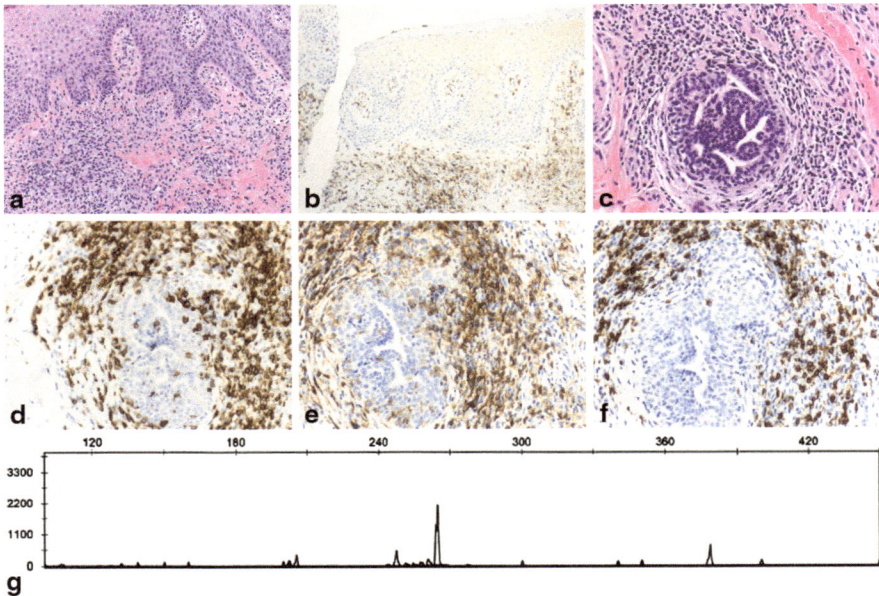

Fig. 2.6 Syringotropic mycosis fungoides. **a** The lesion shows a dermal infiltrate composed of small lymphocytes with mild cytologic atypia. No epidermotropism is seen. Acute inflammation with intraepidermal neutrophils makes the interpretation more cumbersome (H&E, 10x). **b** An immunohistochemical study for CD4 highlights only rare small intraepidermal cells (immunoperoxidase, 10x). **c** Deep dermal lymphocytic infiltrate around eccrine coils. Some hyperchromatic lymphocytes are seen within the adnexal epithelium (H&E, 20x). **d** A CD3 study highlights the syringotropic T lymphocytes (immunoperoxidase, 20x). **e** The syringotropic cells express CD4 (immunoperoxidase, 20x). **f** Numerous CD8-positive T cells are present within the pero-eccrine infiltrate, a confounding finding that may lead to the wrong diagnosis (immunoperoxidase, 20x). **g** *TCR* beta chain gene rearrangement analysis reveals a monoclonal peak in a polyclonal background, supporting the diagnosis of syringotropic mycosis fungoides

Case

A 38-year-old male presented with multiple papules on chest, neck, and upper extremities. Some of the lesions were crusted with pustule formation. The lesions failed to improve on multiple antibiotic and topical treatments. A biopsy demonstrated dermal lymphocytic infiltrate with minimal epidermotropism. Acute inflammation was present in superficial dermis and epidermis. A dense infiltrate was identified around eccrine coils. This infiltrate was demonstrated to be CD3-positive with some CD4-positive cells involving adnexal structures. Numerous CD8-positive cells were also present. Molecular studies for TCR gamma chain gene rearrangement revealed a clonal peak. A diagnosis of syringotropic mycosis fungoides was made (Fig. 2.6) .

Comment: Syringotropic mycosis fungoides may be challenging to diagnose in both clinical and histopathological grounds. The lesions seen in this variant of mycosis fungoides are usually multiple papules or nodules, sometimes associated with anhidrosis [96]. Patches or plaques of typical mycosis fungoides are not usually seen. On histology, careful examination is needed to identify the syringotropic cells. In this case, the associated reactive infiltrate composed of neutrophils and reactive CD8-positive T lymphocytes makes the interpretation of the histopathological findings even more difficult. Demonstration of clonality by *TCR* gene rearrangement studies, along with an adequate interpretation of the pathological and clinical findings, is useful to support a diagnosis of mycosis fungoides in this case. The patient was treated with total skin electron beam therapy with good clinical response.

B-cell Lymphoid Proliferations of the Skin

Primary cutaneous B-cell lymphomas (PCBCL) are B-cell lymphomas originating in the skin with no evidence of extracutaneous disease at the time of diagnosis. The following categories are recognized by the WHO-EORTC (the World Health Organization and the European Organization for Research and Treatment of Cancer) [66, 97]:

1. Primary cutaneous marginal zone B-cell lymphoma (PCMZL)
2. Primary cutaneous follicle centre lymphoma (PCFCL)
3. Primary cutaneous diffuse large B-cell lymphoma, leg type (PCDLBCL, LT)
4. Primary cutaneous diffuse large B-cell lymphoma, other (PCDLBCL, other)

Besides PCBCL, the skin can be secondarily involved by a variety of nodal or systemic B-cell lymphomas. In fact, the skin is the second most common site of extranodal non-Hodgkin lymphoma following the gastrointestinal tract, with an estimated annual incidence of 1:100,000. Although the different types of PCBCL are histologically similar to their corresponding nodal or systemic counterparts, their clinical behavior and prognosis are often different. For example, nodal diffuse large B-cell lymphoma is considered more aggressive compared to primary cutaneous diffuse large B-cell lymphoma. Therefore, it is crucial to recognize and diagnose PCBCL as separate from nodal or systemic B-cell lymphoma secondarily involving the skin.

Here we discuss the 3 main types of PCBCL: PCMZL, PCFCL, and PCDLBCL, LT, and their differential diagnoses with focus on the utility of molecular testing.

Primary Cutaneous Marginal Zone B-cell Lymphoma

Primary cutaneous marginal zone B-cell lymphoma (PCMZL) is an indolent tumor with almost 100% 5-year survival [66]. It is composed of small B-cells including marginal zone (centrocyte-like) cells, lymphoplasmacytoid cells, and plasma cells.

It is considered a part of the broader mucosa-associated lymphoid tissue (MALT) type lymphomas. It affects adults over 40 years and presents as red to violaceous papules, plaques, or nodules, predominantly on the upper extremities and less often on head and trunk.

Histologically, PCMZL is characterized by nodular to diffuse cellular infiltrate with residual reactive lymphoid follicles. The infiltrating cells comprise predominantly centrocyte-like cells or monocytoid cells of small to medium size with slightly irregular nuclei, moderately dispersed chromatin, inconspicuous nucleoli, and moderately abundant pale cytoplasm. These cells are admixed with variable numbers of lymphoplasmacytoid cells and plasma cells, small numbers of centroblasts and numerous reactive T-cells. Intranuclear (Dutcher bodies) or intracytoplasmic periodic acid-schiff (PAS)-positive inclusions may be present, particularly in cases with predominance of lymphoplasmacytoid cells. Diffuse infiltration involving epithelium and sweat glands and the presence of very immature plasma cells suggests secondary involvement by a systemic lymphoma [98].

Immunophenotypically, the neoplastic lymphocytes express B-cell markers CD19, CD20, CD22, and CD79a, and are negative for CD5, CD10, and CD23. In addition, the neoplastic lymphocytes are BCL2 positive and BCL6 negative. The dendritic cell marker CD21 highlights residual or distorted follicular dendritic cell meshworks, where only rare or absent CD10+ or BCL6+ residual germinal center cells may be found; however, most cells in the infiltrate are CD10− and BCL6−. The lymphoplasmacytoid cells and the plasma cells show monotypic cytoplasmic immunoglobulin light chain expression [99]. If evidence of clonality by light chain restriction is demonstrated by immunohistochemistry, there is no compelling need of performing molecular analysis to demonstrate clonality.

Immunoglobulin heavy chain (*IGH*) gene rearrangement studies show monoclonal rearrangements in most cases, in the range of 60 % using one set of FR primers, and almost 100 % using three sets of FR primers [23, 100]. Sequence analyses demonstrate somatic hypermutation in the clonally rearranged IGH variable region. Although most cases do not have recurrent chromosomal translocations, a minority of cases show t(14;18)(q32;q21) involving the *IGH* and *MALT1* genes [31] and t(3;14)(p14.1;q32) involving *IGH* and *FOXP1* genes [101]. The t(11;18)(q21;q21) involving the *API2* and *MALT1* genes that frequently occur in non-cutaneous marginal zone lymphoma of MALT does not occur in PCMZL [102]. Gene rearrangement involving BCL10 has not been reported. Gains of chromosome 3 and 18 may be present [31]. *FAS* gene mutations are detected in a minority of cases, similar to MZL of other extranodal sites. Mutations of other genes occur rarely and these include the oncogenes *PIM1*, *PAX5*, *RhoH/TTF*, and *MYC*. Inactivation of the tumor suppressor genes *CDKN2A* and *DAPK* by hypermethylation has been documented. These findings suggest different pathogenetic pathways between PCMZL and extracutaneous marginal zone lymphoma of MALT and thus support their distinct classification. It is of interest that cases of PCMZL in Europe, but not in the USA have been associated with *Borrelia burgdorferi* [97].

Primary Cutaneous Follicle Centre Lymphoma

Primary cutaneous follicle centre lymphoma (PCFCL) is an indolent lymphoma of follicle center B-cells, with a > 95 % 5-year survival [66]. As its indolent behavior, independent of histologic appearance, grading is not recommended for PCFCL. It predominantly affects middle-aged adults, and the sites most frequently affected are trunk, and head and neck regions [103]. It presents as solitary or grouped firm erythematous plaques or nodules. In contrast to PCMZL, multifocal skin lesions are rare.

Histologically, PCFCL shows a spectrum of growth patterns including a follicular, a follicular and diffuse, and a diffuse pattern, with consistent sparing of the epidermis. Follicles are ill-defined with lack of tingible body macrophages and attenuated or absent mantle zones. The abnormal follicles are composed of a mixture of centrocytes, relatively few centroblasts, and many reactive T-cells, enmeshed in a network of follicular dendritic cells. In advanced lesions, the follicular structures are no longer discernible, and the infiltrating cells are generally large centrocytes with variable admixture of centroblasts and immunoblasts.

Immunophenotypically, the neoplastic lymphocytes express B-cell markers, with co-expression of the germinal center marker BCL6. CD10 is detected in cases with follicular growth pattern but is uncommon in cases with diffuse growth pattern. Focal positivity for MUM-1 is possible, although the tumor cells are usually negative [104]. The neoplastic cells are negative for CD5 and CD43. Unlike nodal and secondary follicular lymphomas, PCFCL cells generally do not express or are faintly positive for BCL2. A strong expression of BCL2 suggests secondary skin infiltration. Monotypic immunoglobulins can be detected by flow cytometry or frozen sections but rarely by routine paraffin immunohistochemistry.

Molecular testing reveals monoclonal *IgH* gene rearrangements in 67% of the cases. Somatic hypermutations of the variable *IgH* gene are common, thus the chance of false negatives can be decreased with the use of multiple primers sets [23, 100]. In contrast to systemic follicular lymphoma, PCFCL commonly lack the t(14;18)(q32;q21) or *BCL2* gene rearrangement [105, 106]. Mutations of oncogenes *BCL6, MYC, RhoH/TTF,* and *PAX5* have been reported. Inactivation of the *CDK-N2A* tumor suppressor gene by deletion or promoter hypermethylation is rare [107]. Array-based comparative genomic hybridization (aCGH) and FISH studies may rarely reveal amplification of chromosome region 2p16 (containing the *c-REL* and *BCL11A* genes) [108] and loss of chromosome 14q32 (containing the *IGH* gene) [107].

Primary Cutaneous Diffuse Large B-Cell Lymphoma, Leg Type

Primary cutaneous diffuse large B-cell lymphoma, leg type (PCDLBCL, LT) is a subtype of diffuse large B-cell lymphoma with an aggressive behavior, and histologically is composed of large transformed cells with a diffuse growth pattern.

Primary cutaneous diffuse large B-cell lymphoma, leg type (PCDLBCL, LT) characteristically involves the legs, [109] but sometimes can occur in trunk and rarely in the head. Primary cutaneous diffuse large B-cell lymphoma, leg type (PCDLBCL, LT) predominantly affects elderly females and presents as multiple rapidly growing nodules [110]. In contrast to indolent cutaneous B-cell lymphomas, they more often disseminate to extracutaneous sites and have a poorer prognosis.

Histologically, PCDLBCL, LT, shows a diffuse infiltrate of large cells in the dermis with a destructive growth pattern obliterating adnexal structures and extending into the subcutaneous tissue, with sparing of the epidermis. The infiltrating tumor cells monotonous population or confluent sheets of centroblasts and immunoblasts [111]. Mitotic figures are frequently observed.

Immunophenotypically, the neoplastic lymphocytes express B-cell markers, and light chain restriction can be demonstrated by flow cytometry immunophenotype or frozen section, but no paraffin section immunohistochemistry. The neoplastic cells commonly express BCL2 and IRF4/MUM1 [112, 113]. They variably express BCL6 and generally do not express CD10.

Molecular testing reveals monoclonal *IgH* gene rearrangements in almost 100 % of cases [23]. The t(14;18) involving the *BCL2* gene is usually not present [114], however, cases with gene amplification of BCL2 have been reported [115]. Gene expression profiling studies showed gene expression profile similar to that of activated B-cell type of nodal or systemic DLBCL [116]. Array-based comparative genomic hybridization (aCGH) and FISH studies showed frequent deletion of chromosome 9p21 (containing the *CDKN2A* and *CDKN2B* genes) and amplification of 18q21 (containing the *BCL2* and *MALT1* genes). Other chromosomal aberrations include gains in chromosomes 1, 2, 3, 7, 12, and 18q, and losses in 6q, 13, and 17 [108]. Inactivation of CDKN2A by promoter hypermethylation is also detected. The inactivation of CDKN2A, either by deletion or promoter hypermethylation is a poor prognostic marker [107].

Case

A 54-year-old male presented with nodules in the scalp. The patient did not have a significant medical history. On physical examination, scalp nodules, less than 1 cm in diameter were palpated, and a punch biopsy was obtained. The histologic sections showed a dense dermal infiltrate without epidermal involvement. There were scattered lymphoid follicles with germinal center formation. Immunohistochemical studies showed the lymphoid follicles to react with B-cell markers CD20 and PAX-5. BCL2 was negative in the germinal centers (Fig. 2.7 a and b).

Comment: The differential diagnosis is between follicular lymphoid hyperplasia and primary cutaneous follicular lymphoma. Molecular testing for *IGH* gene rearrangements yielded a polyclonal pattern, thus it failed to detected monoclonality. However, because of the possibility of follicular lymphoma, testing for t(14:18) (q32;q21) *IGH/BCL2* by PCR was performed and demonstrated the presence of the

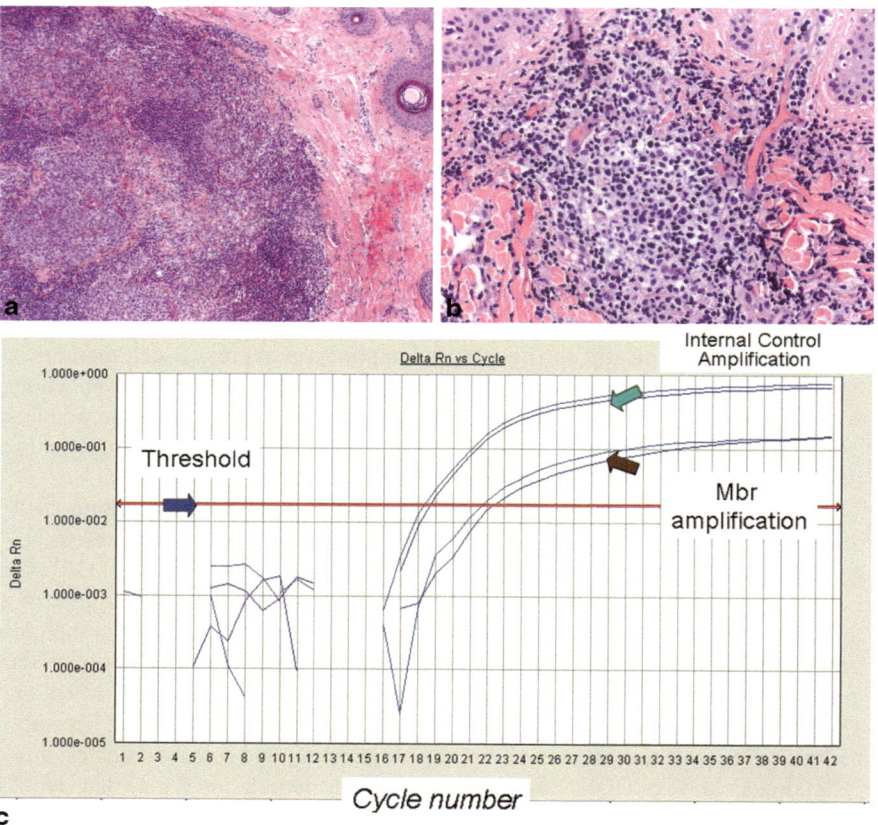

c

Fig. 2.7 Primary cutaneous follicle centre lymphoma harboring the t(14:18)(q32;q21) *IGH/BCL2* translocation. **a** The skin biopsy shows a dense dermal infiltrate with ill defined follicles with germinal centers (H&E, 10x). **b** The germinal centers are composed of a mixture of centrocytes, centroblasts, and many reactive small lymphocytes (H&E, 20x) **c** Molecular analysis for *IGH-BCL2* rearrangement associated with the t(14;18)(q32;q21.3) was performed by real-time PCR using specific primers that target the major breakpoint region (mbr) of the *BCL2* gene. Amplification of the cyclophilin gene is used as an internal control for sample adequacy for PCR. *IGH* gene rearrangement analysis revealed a polyclonal pattern (not shown). Although the presence of *IGH-BCL2* translocation should raise suspicion for systemic follicular lymphoma with secondary involvement of the skin, the clinical workup in this patient was negative for systemic disease and a diagnosis of primary cutaneous follicle centre lymphoma was favored

rearrangement (Fig. 2.7c). This rearrangement is commonly associated with nodal follicular lymphoma, but it can also be present in some primary cutaneous follicular lymphomas, as illustrated in this case. On follow up, clinical staging was negative, and the disease was confined to the scalp. Local radiation, but no systemic therapy was administered, and the patient was asymptomatic on last follow up 5 years after diagnosis.

Leukemia Cutis

Leukemia cutis (LC) is an all encompassing term which describes a neoplastic infiltrate of the skin by myeloid (granulocytic or monocytic) or lymphoid precursor cells. LC composed of myeloid blast with granulocytic differentiation may also be designated as chloroma, granulocytic sarcoma, extramedullary myeloid sarcoma and monoblastic sarcoma if precursor cells demonstrate monoblast or promonocytic differentiation [117, 118]. LC may be present in the context of known myeloid or lymphoid disorders or may present as aleukemic LC in patients with no prior history of a hematologic malignancy. Aleukemic LC occurs in majority of cases which demonstrate myelomonocytic or monocytic differentiation [119–121].

Molecular analysis of LC lesions has been reported for a variety of hematopoietic malignancy including AML, acute promyelocytic leukemia, and mature T-cell leukemias [122–126]. Although, genetic abnormalities in LC lesions appear to be concordant with testing in bone marrow there are some exceptions and molecular testing may be beneficial in aleukemic LC, particularly if the infiltrate is composed of myeloid blasts since recurring genetic abnormalities defines some categories of AML classification. The 2008 World Health Organization (WHO) classification scheme of AML incorporates clinical, immunophenotypic and cytogenetic features which classifies AML in four main categories: (1) AML with recurrent genetic abnormalities, (2) AML with myelodysplasia related changes, (3) AML related to therapy, and (4) AML not otherwise specified [117]. Recurring genetic abnormalities in patients with AML and manifestation of LC include *NPM1* mutations, inv (16), abnormalities in chromosome 8 copy number, *MLL* (11q23) gene rearrangement [127–130]. Evaluation of genetic abnormalities in LC may aid may confirm and/or establish diagnosis in aleukemic patients as well as allow for evaluation of concordant genetic abnormalities in skin and bone marrow lesions [126].

Clinically, LC may present as a solitary or multiple violaceous, hemorrhagic papules, nodule or plaques with propensity for extremities, although any part of the body can be affected [131]. Histologically, the pattern of infiltrate may be perivascular and periadnexal or diffuse with infiltrate of single cells between collagen bundles or concentric layering around blood vessels and adnexal structures [132]. Further, lineage classification of the tumor cells will require cytochemical and/or immunohistochemical analysis.

Leukemic infiltrate in the skin may be secondarily involved in reactive inflammatory processes and may be misinterpreted as LC. For example, patient's with CLL/SLL often demonstrate an exuberant hypersensitivity reaction to arthropod bite and histologic examination of the lesion will demonstrate circulating leukemic cells which has secondarily involved the skin from damaged or permeable vessels [133]. The diagnosis of LC would be inappropriate in this clinical setting.

Reactive Lymphoid Proliferations

There is a spectrum of reactive lymphoid proliferations in the skin that may mimic cutaneous T- or B-cell lymphomas both clinically and histologically. The etiology of these reactive lymphoid proliferations or "pseudolymphomas" varies with majority of the lesion being idiopathic. Some of the lymphoid reactions may be secondary to foreign antigens, medications, infection, and connective tissue disorders and can present clinically and histologically as contact dermatitis, drug reactions, secondary syphilis, arthropod assault, lichen sclerosus, morphea, and lupus panniculitis [134].

The distinction from benign and malignant lymphoid proliferations of the skin is one of the challenges in dermatopathology and requires analysis of the all the clinical, histologic, immunohistochemcial, and molecular features that are available to arrive at the accurate diagnosis. However, even with integration of all available studies, in some cases the accurate diagnosis will not become apparent until after years of clinical follow up [135].

The identification of a monoclonal T- or B-cell population in a lymphoid infiltrate of the skin by PCR analysis of gamma and beta chains of TCR or the immunoglobulin heavy chain (JH) aids in the distinction between benign and malignant T- and B-cell proliferations, respectively. Clonality however does not necessarily imply malignancy. Pseudoclonality or the detection of a single clonal T- or B-cell population that are of different size on repeat analysis have been described in reactive lymphoid conditions of the skin including, lichen planus, eythema chronicum migrans, pityriasis lichenoides, lymphomatoid keratosis, varicella zoster virus induced folliculitis and cutaneous lymphoid hyperplasia [136–140]. In fact, the detection of T and B pseudoclones was reported in 13 and 23 % of reactive infiltrates of the skin, respectively. There was greater likelihood of T- or B-cell pseudoclone detection in cases of moderately dense lymphoid infiltrates and many of the B-cell pseudoclones were identified in cases which contained sparse population of B-cell [141]. Many of the inflammatory dermatoses of the skin demonstrate a T-cell infiltrate composed of a mixed population of CD4 and CD8 positive T cells. There are some dermatologic entities that... CD20 positive cells and are positive for the presence of pseudoclones, which may simuate cutaneous lymphoma. These conditions will be further discussed in the paragraphs below.

Lymphomatoid contact dermatitis may simulate MF and have been described in association with gold, nickel, phenol resin, and wood species of Teak [142–145]. Lesions may clinically manifest as recurrent erythematous plaques and histologically demonstrate a dense lymphoid infiltrate in the dermis with variable degree of spongiosis in the epidermis with vesiculation. The lymphocytic infiltrate is predominantly composed of CD3 and CD4 positive T cells with scattered eosinophils in the biopsy. CD7 expression may be variable and decreased in reactive conditions as well as in MF [40]. At times, an intraepidermal mononuclear cell collection (intraepidermal microgranulomas or pseudo Pautrier microabscesses) may be encountered and are composed of CD1a and S100 positive cells [146, 147]. T-cell receptor (*TCR*) gene rearrangement studies typically demonstrate a polyclonal T-cell infiltrate; however, clonal *T-cell* gene rearrangement do occur in this setting and bears no clinical significance[148].

Parapsoriasis is a chronic persistent skin eruption with fine scales is and can clinically and histologically simulate mycosis fungoides and certain clinical subtypes of parapsoriasis (e.g., large plaque parapsoriasis or parapsoriasis en plaque) may be biologically related to mycosis fungoides [149]. The clinical subtypes of parapsoriasis initially described by Brocq include: (1) small plaque (French word "plaque" is equivalent to patch) parapsoriasis (SPP) and (2) large plaque parapsoriasis (LPP) (parapsoriasis en plaques). Both SPP and LPP may demonstrate clonal *T-cell* gene rearrangement and may progress to MF. Large plaque parapsoriasis clinically appear similar to features of MF with patches greater than 6.0 cm in size on non-sun exposed areas. Large plaque parapsoriasis (LPP) may progress to mycosis fungoides in 10–46 % and cases and distinction from LPP and MF may be arbitrary since both terms may refer to the same clinical disease [149, 151].

Small plaque parapsoriasis (or digitate dermatosis, xanthoerythroderma perstans, chronic superficial dermatosis) is clinically characterized by patches 2.0–6.0 cm in size and preferentially located on the lateral aspects of the trunks. A study by Burg et al. examined 82 patients with clinical features of SPP and after over 5–35 years none of the patients progressed to MF [152]. However, examination of 69 patients with SPP by Vakeva et al. demonstrated 7 (10 %) of patients progressed to MF over a medium time of 10 years [153]. SPP appears a distinct entity from MF based on the uniform appearance of small patches with yellow hue, unlikely transformation to MF, and occasional detection of T-cell clonality. Small plaque parapsoriasis (SPP) may be considered an abortive lymphoma and the neoplastic T-cell clone, if present in SPP, appears to be held in check by host control mechanisms and if overcome progression to lymphoma may develop [152].

Pityriasis lichenoides is a chronic, recurrent papulosquamous to papulonecrotic skin disorder. There are two clinical subtype. Pityriasis lichenoides et varioliformis acuta (PLEVA) or Mucha-Habermann disease and pityriasis lichenoides chronica (PLC). Pityriasis lichenoides et varioliformis acuta (PLEVA) is typically seen in children and clinically presents as crops of recurrent papules, which spontaneously regress leaving varioliform scars [154]. Pityriasis lichenoides chronica (PLC) more often is seen in the third decade of life and clinically appears as papule with red brown color and mica-like scales. Lesions will regress over few weeks and leave a hypo or hyperpigmented macule. Histologically PLEVA and PLC demonstrate a dense dermal lichenoid lymphocytic infiltrate with variable degree of keratinocyte injury and necrosis of epidermis in PLEVA and scattered dyskeratotic cells in PLC. The lymphocytic infiltrate is a mixture of CD4 and CD8 positive T cells. CD8 positive cells may be a predominant epidermal component in PLEVA whereas CD4 positive T cells predominate in PLC. Loss of CD7 may be observed and T-cell clonality may be seen in a majority of the cases. In one series, greater than 90 % of the cases analyzed demonstrated clonal T cell with variable detection of clonality in PLEVA (up to 65 %) and PLC (8–50 %) [138, 155, 156].

Pigmented purpuric dermatosis is a chronic dermatologic disorder with different clinical subtypes, which include purpura annularis telangiectodes of Majocchi, progressive pigmentary dermatosis of Schamberg, lichenoid purpura of Gougerot-Blum, eczematoid-like purpura of Doucas and Kapetanakis, and lichen aureus. Lesions typical occur in the lower extremities as multiple red to brown patches, papules or plaques (or single annular patch in the case of lichen aureus) with variable degree of petechia and eczematous scale depending on the clinical subtype [157]. Histologically there is a moderate superficial perivascular or band like lymphoid infiltrate admixed with siderophages and dermal red blood cell extravasation. Immunohistochemically, there is a predominance of CD4 positive T cells over CD8 positive T cells in the infiltrate with loss of CD7 staining [158].

Lichenoid purpura of Gougerot-Blum and lichen aureus have been reported to demonstrate clonal TCR and have been speculated to be biologically related to MF, especially in cases were identical T cell clones were identified in different biopsy samples [159, 160]. However, in 23 patients with classic clinical and histologic features of lichen aureus including 8 cases with monoclonality, there was no progression to MF after mean follow up of 102.1 months [161]. Some cases of PPD demonstrated progression to MF and the distinction from clonal PPD to purpuric MF is heavily dependent on the clinical features which may justify by some authors to categorize clonal PPD as a form of chronic lymphoid dyscrasia [158].

Lupus erythematosus panniculitis (LEP) or lupus profundus is a reactive lymphoid condition involving the subcutaneous tissue of the skin which can simulate subcutaneous panniculitis like T cell lymphoma (SPTCL). Lupus erythematosus panniculitis (LEP) occurs in 1–3 % of patients with cutaneous lupus erythematosus and may be associated with other skin manifestations of LE [162]. Diagnosis of LEP becomes especially challenging when LEP is an isolated finding with or without systemic features and clinical distinction from LEP and SPTCL is not apparent.

Histologically, LEP is a reactive lobular and septal panniculitis composed of lymphoid infiltrate involving the lobules and septate of subcutaneous tissue composed of mixed population of CD4 and CD8 positive cells with more predominance of CD4 compared with CD8 in contrast to SPTCL which is a lymphoma of CD8 positive cytotoxic T cells. Septal fibrosis, hyaline necrosis, B-cell lymphoid aggregates with germinal center formation and plasma cell infiltrate define LEP and absence of prominent cytotoxic CD8 cells with significant atypia will further aid in the distinction from LEP from SPTCL [163, 164]. Rimming of fat lobules may be seen in LEP and SPTCL; however with LEP rimming was by mix population of lymphocytes, plasma cells and histiocytes [163]. Greater than 90 % of LEP typically demonstrates polyclonal TCR and cases with atypical clinical and histologic features may display clonality, although disease progression to lymphoma was not observed [163–165]. Clonal T cells in panniculitis have been described; however, clonality does not necessarily imply lymphoma and may represent a clonal T-cell dyscrasia reported as atypical lymphocytic lobular panniculitis [166].

Vitiligo is a pigmentary disorder which primarily affects the skin and presents clinically as hypopigmented patches. Vitiligo may clinically and histologically simulate hypopigmented MF and both disorders demonstrate a loss of melanocytes in the epidermis [167]. Biopsy of an inflammatory lesion of vitiligo will demonstrate band like infiltrate of lymphocytes in the dermis with lymphocytic exocytosis.

Immunohistochemically the lymphoid infiltrate is composed of CD8 cytotoxic T cells. Hypopigmented MF also demonstrates epidermotropic CD8 positive lymphocytes. T cell analysis will aid in the distinction since cases of vitiligo demonstrate polyclonal TCR [168].

Infectious processes, arthropod assaults and drug reactions may demonstrate an ulcerative necrotic papule or nodule with increase number of CD30 positive lymphocytes which resemble CD30 positive lymphoproliferative disorder [169, 170]. Clinical history and analysis of *TCR* gene rearrangement or viral DNA will enable to further distinguish these reactive CD30 lymphoid proliferations from lymphoma since the reactive disorder will demonstrate polyclonal TCR and viral DNA may identify the infectious organism.

Cutaneous lymphoid hyperplasia (CLH) or lymphocytoma cutis is a reactive proliferation seen primarily on the head and neck as a solitary brown purple nodule. Cutaneous lymphoid hyperplasia (CLH) may also clinically present as groups of papules or nodules and less frequently widely scattered on the body. Multiple lesions and features of recurrence which may be seen in CLH make distinction from lymphoma a diagnostic challenge. Cutaneous lymphoid hyperplasia (CLH) may be idiopathic or may be seen in response to arthropod bite, *B. burgdorferi* infection, vaccination, drugs, and other foreign antigenic stimulation [171].

Histologically, CLH may have well to ill-defined lymphoid follicles or germinal centers or may be a diffuse, nodular proliferation with absence of lymphoid follicles. Immunohistochemically CLH may be composed of either a predominance of T or B cells, but often will demonstrate a mixed lymphohistiocytic population admixed with plasma cells. Reactive lymphoid follicles will be positive for CD20, CD10, BCL6, and demonstrate increase proliferative rate with Ki-67 and negative for BCL2. Anti-CD21 is a marker which will highlight the dendritic meshwork of a germinal center which may help highlight lesions with ill-defined lymphoid follicles. CD3 positive T cells will be distributed between the lymphoid follicles and as single cells within the lymphoid follicles. Lesions with absence of lymphoid follicles will demonstrate mixture of T and B cells. The B cells may be in aggregates and are negative for BCL6, CD10, and BCL2. CD21 will also be negative since lymphoid follicles are absent. Variable numbers of polytypic kappa and lambda positive plasma cells are usually within the reactive lymphoid infiltrate [172].

Molecular analysis of immunoglobulin heavy chain (JH) in CLH is typically polyclonal; however, B-cell clonality in CLH is known to occur and in one series up to 41 % of the cases demonstrated clonal B-cell population [173]. Clonality did not correlate with clinical and morphologic features of lymphoma. Cutaneous lymphoid hyperplasia (CLH) may simulate follicular lymphoma and marginal zone lymphoma. In the skin, marginal zone lymphoma (MZL) is a main differential diagnosis of CLH since MZL often demonstrates reactive appearing areas. The presence of monotypic plasma cell population along with the other clinical, histologic, immunohistochemcial, and molecular features may aid in distinction of MZL from CLH.

Lymphomatoid drug reactions may be caused by a variety of agents including anticonvulsants, antidepressants, angiotensin-converting enzyme inhibitors, histamine receptor antagonists, and targeted therapy with monoclonal antibodies (MAB)

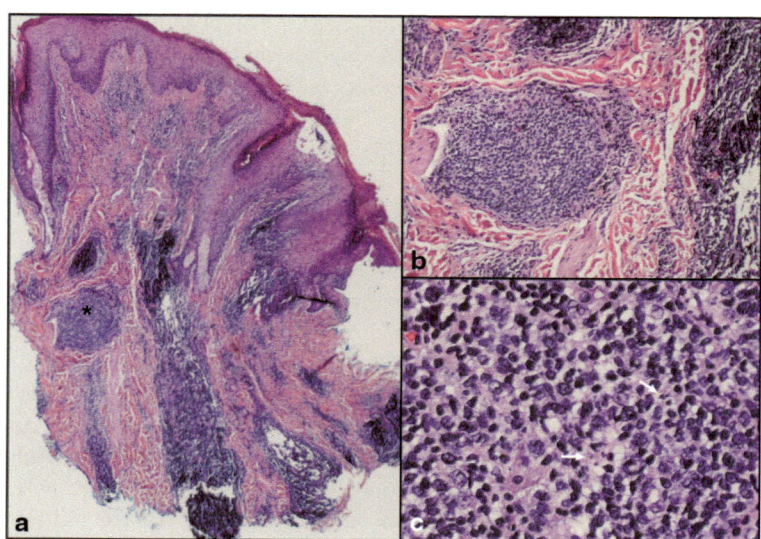

Fig. 2.8 a Skin punch with lymphocytic infiltrate in the dermis in a periadnexal and perivascular distribution with lymphoid follicle formation (*). **b** and **c** Reactive lymphoid follicle in dermis with centrocytes and tingle body macrophages (*arrows*)

which can clinically and histologically mimic cutaneous T cell lymphoma, B-cell lymphoma, and CD30 positive lymphoproliferative disorders [174–176]. Lesion will regress if the causative agent is removed and molecular analysis typically demonstrates a polyclonal pattern. In some instances, lymphomatoid drug reactions may demonstrate morphologic atypia, clonality and loss of CD7 and or CD62K and may represent drug induced clonal expansion of these subset of lymphocytes [176].

Case

A 58-year-old white male presented with 3 year history of multiple plaques and nodules on the forehead ranging in measurement from 2.0 to 3.0 cm. A representative biopsy of the forehead lesion demonstrated a nodular dermal lymphocytic infiltrate with reactive lymphoid follicles with tingible body macrophages and centrocytes. Mature small lymphocytes admixed with histiocytes and plasma cells were seen between the reactive lymphoid follicles and in a periadnexal pattern (Fig. 2.8). Immunohistochemically, the infiltrate is primary CD3 positive with cells in the reactive lymphoid follicle positive for CD20, BCL6, and negative for BCL2. Kappa and lambda in situ hybridization fails to detect monotypic plasma cell population and *IgH* gene rearrangement was not identified (Fig. 2.9).

Comment: The diagnosis is cutaneous lymphoid hyperplasia with formation of reactive germinal centers. Systemic workup has been negative for lymphoma and

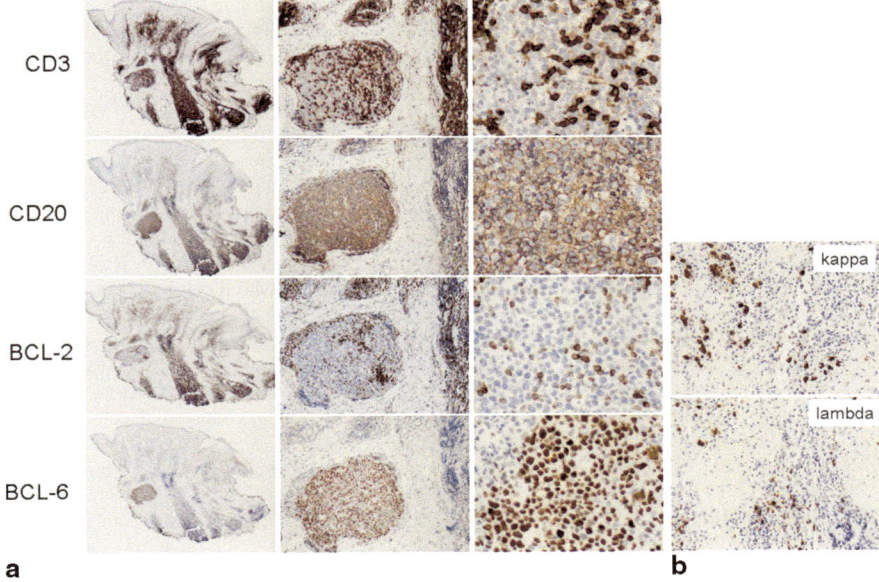

a   b

Fig. 2.9 a Immunohistochemical analysis with anti-CD3, CD20, BCL2, BCL6. Lymphoid infiltrate composed of CD3 and CD20 positive lymphocytes with reactive lymphoid follicle composed of CD20 positive B cells with few intrafollicular CD3 reactive T cells (*top* two rows). CD20 positive B cells in the reactive lymphoid follicle are negative for BCL2 and positive for BCL6 (*bottom* two rows). **b** Polytypic pattern of kappa and lambda plasma cells by in situ hybridization

B. burgdorferi titers are negative. Therapy with topical and intralesional steroids and cryotherapy have been unsuccessful and patient is currently managed with palliative radiation. Radiation therapy may become a treatment option in CLH cases refractory to steroid or cyrotherapy.

References

1. Sandberg Y, Heule F, Lam K, et al. Molecular immunoglobulin/T-cell receptor clonality analysis in cutaneous lymphoproliferations. Experience with the BIOMED-2 standardized polymerase chain reaction protocol. Haematologica. 2003;88(6):659–70.
2. Winoto A, Baltimore D. Alpha beta lineage-specific expression of the alpha T cell receptor gene by nearby silencers. Cell. 1989;59(4):649–55.
3. Groenen PJ, Langerak AW, van Dongen JJ, van Krieken JH. Pitfalls in TCR gene clonality testing: teaching cases. J Hematop. 2008;1(2):97–109.
4. Theodorou I, Raphael M, Bigorgne C, et al. Recombination pattern of the *TCR* gamma locus in human peripheral T-cell lymphomas. J Pathol. 1994;174(4):233–42.
5. Baer R, Boehm T, Yssel H, Spits H, Rabbitts TH. Complex rearrangements within the human J delta-C delta/J alpha-C alpha locus and aberrant recombination between J alpha segments. EMBO J. 1988;7(6):1661–8.

6. van Dongen JJ, Langerak AW, Bruggemann M, et al. Design and standardization of PCR primers and protocols for detection of clonal immunoglobulin and T-cell receptor gene recombinations in suspect lymphoproliferations: report of the BIOMED-2 Concerted Action BMH4-CT98-3936. Leukemia. 2003;17(12):2257–317.
7. Trainor KJ, Brisco MJ, Wan JH, Neoh S, Grist S, Morley AA. Gene rearrangement in B- and T-lymphoproliferative disease detected by the polymerase chain reaction. Blood. 1991;78(1):192–6.
8. Assaf C, Hummel M, Steinhoff M, et al. Early TCR-beta and TCR-gamma PCR detection of T-cell clonality indicates minimal tumor disease in lymph nodes of cutaneous T-cell lymphoma: diagnostic and prognostic implications. Blood. 2005;105(2):503–10.
9. van Krieken JH, Elwood L, Andrade RE, Jaffe ES, Cossman J, Medeiros LJ. Rearrangement of the T-cell receptor delta chain gene in T-cell lymphomas with a mature phenotype. Am J Pathol. 1991;139(1):161–8.
10. Sprouse JT, Werling R, Hanke D, et al. T-cell clonality determination using polymerase chain reaction (PCR) amplification of the T-cell receptor gamma-chain gene and capillary electrophoresis of fluorescently labeled PCR products. Am J Clin Pathol. 2000;113(6):838–50.
11. Wood GS, Greenberg HL. Diagnosis, staging, and monitoring of cutaneous T-cell lymphoma. Dermatol Ther. 2003;16(4):269–75.
12. Meyerson HJ. Flow cytometry for the diagnosis of mycosis fungoides. G Ital Dermatol Venereol. 2008;143(1):21–41.
13. Weiss LM, Picker LJ, Grogan TM, Warnke RA, Sklar J. Absence of clonal beta and gamma T-cell receptor gene rearrangements in a subset of peripheral T-cell lymphomas. Am J Pathol. 1988;130(3):436–42.
14. Ponti R, Fierro MT, Quaglino P, et al. TCRgamma-chain gene rearrangement by PCR-based GeneScan: diagnostic accuracy improvement and clonal heterogeneity analysis in multiple cutaneous T-cell lymphoma samples. J Invest Dermatol. 2008;128(4):1030–8.
15. Klemke CD, Poenitz N, Dippel E, Hummel M, Stein H, Goerdt S. T-cell clonality of undetermined significance. Arch Dermatol. 2006;142(3):393–4.
16. Thurber SE, Zhang B, Kim YH, Schrijver I, Zehnder J, Kohler S. T-cell clonality analysis in biopsy specimens from two different skin sites shows high specificity in the diagnosis of patients with suggested mycosis fungoides. J Am Acad Dermatol. 2007;57(5):782–90.
17. Guitart J, Magro C. Cutaneous T-cell lymphoid dyscrasia: a unifying term for idiopathic chronic dermatoses with persistent T-cell clones. Arch Dermatol. 2007;143(7):921–32.
18. Rubben A, Kempf W, Kadin ME, Zimmermann DR, Burg G. Multilineage progression of genetically unstable tumor subclones in cutaneous T-cell lymphoma. Exp Dermatol. 2004;13(8):472–83.
19. Bignon YJ, Souteyrand P, Roger H, et al. Clonotypic heterogeneity in cutaneous T-cell lymphomas. Cancer Res. 1990;50(20):6620–5.
20. Vega F, Luthra R, Medeiros LJ, et al. Clonal heterogeneity in mycosis fungoides and its relationship to clinical course. Blood. 2002;100(9):3369–73.
21. Alt FW, Yancopoulos GD, Blackwell TK, et al. Ordered rearrangement of immunoglobulin heavy chain variable region segments. EMBO J. 1984;3(6):1209–19.
22. Wan JH, Trainor KJ, Brisco MJ, Morley AA. Monoclonality in B cell lymphoma detected in paraffin wax embedded sections using the polymerase chain reaction. J Clin Pathol. 1990;43(11):888–90.
23. Lukowsky A, Marchwat M, Sterry W, Gellrich S. Evaluation of B-cell clonality in archival skin biopsy samples of cutaneous B-cell lymphoma by immunoglobulin heavy chain gene polymerase chain reaction. Leuk Lymphoma. 2006;47(3):487–93.
24. Derksen PW, Langerak AW, Kerkhof E, et al. Comparison of different polymerase chain reaction-based approaches for clonality assessment of immunoglobulin heavy-chain gene rearrangements in B-cell neoplasia. Mod Pathol. 1999;12(8):794–805.
25. Gong JZ, Zheng S, Chiarle R, et al. Detection of immunoglobulin kappa light chain rearrangements by polymerase chain reaction. An improved method for detecting clonal B-cell lymphoproliferative disorders. Am J Pathol. 1999;155(2):355–63.

26. Nihal M, Mikkola D, Horvath N, et al. Cutaneous lymphoid hyperplasia: a lymphoprolifera-tive continuum with lymphomatous potential. Hum Pathol. 2003;34(6):617–22.
27. Pilozzi E, Muller-Hermelink HK, Falini B, et al. Gene rearrangements in T-cell lymphoblas-tic lymphoma. J Pathol. 1999;188(3):267–70.
28. Iqbal J, Sanger WG, Horsman DE, et al. BCL2 translocation defines a unique tumor sub-set within the germinal center B-cell-like diffuse large B-cell lymphoma. Am J Pathol. 2004;165(1):159–66.
29. Weiss LM, Warnke RA, Sklar J, Cleary ML. Molecular analysis of the t(14;18) chromosomal translocation in malignant lymphomas. N Engl J Med. 1987;317(19):1185–9.
30. Mirza I, Macpherson N, Paproski S, et al. Primary cutaneous follicular lymphoma: an assess-ment of clinical, histopathologic, immunophenotypic, and molecular features. J Clin Oncol. 2002;20(3):647–55.
31. Streubel B, Lamprecht A, Dierlamm J, et al. T(14;18)(q32;q21) involving IGH and MALT1 is a frequent chromosomal aberration in MALT lymphoma. Blood. 2003;101(6):2335–9.
32. Morris SW, Kirstein MN, Valentine MB, et al. Fusion of a kinase gene, ALK, to a nucleolar protein gene, NPM, in non-Hodgkin's lymphoma. Science. 1994;263(5151):1281–4.
33. Gould JW, Eppes RB, Gilliam AC, et al. Solitary primary cutaneous CD30+ large cell lym-phoma of natural killer cell phenotype bearing the t(2;5)(p23;q35) translocation and present-ing in a child. Am J Dermatopathol. 2000;22(5):422–8.
34. Chuang SS, Hsieh YC, Ye H, Hwang WS. Lymphohistiocytic anaplastic large cell lymphoma involving skin: a diagnostic challenge. Pathol Res Pract. 2009;205(4):283–7.
35. Wada DA, Law ME, Hsi ED, et al. Specificity of IRF4 translocations for primary cutane-ous anaplastic large cell lymphoma: a multicenter study of 204 skin biopsies. Mod Pathol. 2011;24(4):596–605.
36. Weiss LM, Movahed LA, Chen YY, et al. Detection of immunoglobulin light-chain mRNA in lymphoid tissues using a practical in situ hybridization method. Am J Pathol. 1990;137(4):979–88.
37. Herbst H, Steinbrecher E, Niedobitek G, et al. Distribution and phenotype of Epstein-Barr virus-harboring cells in Hodgkin's disease. Blood. 1992;80(2):484–91.
38. Pimpinelli N, Olsen EA, Santucci M, et al. Defining early mycosis fungoides. J Am Acad Dermatol. 2005;53(6):1053–63.
39. Zinzani PL, Ferreri AJ, Cerroni L. Mycosis fungoides. Crit Rev Oncol Hematol. 2008;65(2):172–82.
40. Murphy M, Fullen D, Carlson JA. Low CD7 expression in benign and malignant cutaneous lymphocytic infiltrates: experience with an antibody reactive with paraffin-embedded tissue. Am J Dermatopathol. 2002;24(1):6–16.
41. Massone C, Crisman G, Kerl H, Cerroni L. The prognosis of early mycosis fungoides is not influenced by phenotype and T-cell clonality. Br J Dermatol. 2008;159(4):881–6.
42. Liebmann RD, Anderson B, McCarthy KP, Chow JW. The polymerase chain reaction in the diagnosis of early mycosis fungoides. J Pathol. 1997;182(3):282–7.
43. Guitart J, Camisa C, Ehrlich M, Bergfeld WF. Long-term implications of T-cell receptor gene rearrangement analysis by Southern blot in patients with cutaneous T-cell lymphoma. J Am Acad Dermatol. 2003;48(5):775–9.
44. Signoretti S, Murphy M, Cangi MG, Puddu P, Kadin ME, Loda M. Detection of clonal T-cell receptor gamma gene rearrangements in paraffin-embedded tissue by polymerase chain reac-tion and nonradioactive single-strand conformational polymorphism analysis. Am J Pathol. 1999;154(1):67–75.
45. Li N, Bhawan J. New insights into the applicability of T-cell receptor gamma gene rearrange-ment analysis in cutaneous T-cell lymphoma. J Cutan Pathol. 2001;28(8):412–8.
46. Olsen EA, Rook AH, Zic J, et al. Sezary syndrome: immunopathogenesis, literature review of therapeutic options, and recommendations for therapy by the United States Cutaneous Lymphoma Consortium (USCLC). J Am Acad Dermatol. 2011;64(2):352–404.

47. Campbell JJ, Clark RA, Watanabe R, Kupper TS. Sezary syndrome and mycosis fungoides arise from distinct T-cell subsets: a biologic rationale for their distinct clinical behaviors. Blood. 2010;116(5):767–71.
48. Diwan AH, Prieto VG, Herling M, Duvic M, Jone D. Primary Sezary syndrome commonly shows low-grade cytologic atypia and an absence of epidermotropism. Am J Clin Pathol. 2005;123(4):510–5.
49. Beylot-Barry M, Sibaud V, Thiebaut R, et al. Evidence that an identical T cell clone in skin and peripheral blood lymphocytes is an independent prognostic factor in primary cutaneous T cell lymphomas. J Invest Dermatol. 2001;117(4):920–6.
50. Delfau-Larue MH, Laroche L, Wechsler J, et al. Diagnostic value of dominant T-cell clones in peripheral blood in 363 patients presenting consecutively with a clinical suspicion of cutaneous lymphoma. Blood. 2000;96(9):2987–92.
51. Dereure O, Balavoine M, Salles MT, et al. Correlations between clinical, histologic, blood, and skin polymerase chain reaction outcome in patients treated for mycosis fungoides. J Invest Dermatol. 2003;121(3):614–7.
52. Willemze R, Beljaards RC. Spectrum of primary cutaneous CD30 (Ki-1)-positive lymphoproliferative disorders. A proposal for classification and guidelines for management and treatment. J Am Acad Dermatol. 1993;28(6):973–80.
53. Bekkenk MW, Geelen FA, van Voorst Vader PC, et al. Primary and secondary cutaneous CD30(+) lymphoproliferative disorders: a report from the Dutch Cutaneous Lymphoma Group on the long-term follow-up data of 219 patients and guidelines for diagnosis and treatment. Blood. 2000;95(12):3653–61.
54. Willemze R, Kerl H, Sterry W, et al. EORTC classification for primary cutaneous lymphomas: a proposal from the cutaneous lymphoma study group of the European organization for research and treatment of cancer. Blood. 1997;90(1):354–71.
55. Saggini A, Gulia A, Argenyi Z, et al. A variant of lymphomatoid papulosis simulating primary cutaneous aggressive epidermotropic CD8+ cytotoxic T-cell lymphoma. Description of 9 cases. Am J Surg Pathol. 2010;34(8):1168–75.
56. Greisser J, Palmedo G, Sander C, et al. Detection of clonal rearrangement of T-cell receptor genes in the diagnosis of primary cutaneous CD30 lymphoproliferative disorders. J Cutan Pathol. 2006;33(11):711–5.
57. Zackheim HS, Jones C, Leboit PE, Kashani-Sabet M, McCalmont TH, Zehnder J. Lymphomatoid papulosis associated with mycosis fungoides: a study of 21 patients including analyses for clonality. J Am Acad Dermatol. 2003;49(4):620–3.
58. Chott A, Vonderheid EC, Olbricht S, Miao NN, Balk SP, Kadin ME. The dominant T cell clone is present in multiple regressing skin lesions and associated T cell lymphomas of patients with lymphomatoid papulosis. J Invest Dermatol. 1996;106(4):696–700.
59. DeCoteau JF, Butmarc JR, Kinney MC, Kadin ME. The t(2;5) chromosomal translocation is not a common feature of primary cutaneous CD30+ lymphoproliferative disorders: comparison with anaplastic large-cell lymphoma of nodal origin. Blood. 1996;87(8):3437–41.
60. Beltraminelli H, Leinweber B, Kerl H, Cerroni L. Primary cutaneous CD4+ small-/medium-sized pleomorphic T-cell lymphoma: a cutaneous nodular proliferation of pleomorphic T lymphocytes of undetermined significance? A study of 136 cases. Am J Dermatopathol. 2009;31(4):317–22.
61. Garcia-Herrera A, Colomo L, Camos M, et al. Primary cutaneous small/medium CD4+ T-cell lymphomas: a heterogeneous group of tumors with different clinicopathologic features and outcome. J Clin Oncol. 2008;26(20):3364–71.
62. Rodriguez Pinilla SM, Roncador G, Rodriguez-Peralto JL, et al. Primary cutaneous CD4+ small/medium-sized pleomorphic T-cell lymphoma expresses follicular T-cell markers. Am J Surg Pathol. 2009;33(1):81–90.
63. Berti E, Tomasini D, Vermeer MH, Meijer CJ, Alessi E, Willemze R. Primary cutaneous CD8-positive epidermotropic cytotoxic T cell lymphomas. A distinct clinicopathological entity with an aggressive clinical behavior. Am J Pathol. 1999;155(2):483–92.

64. Introcaso CE, Kim EJ, Gardner J, Junkins-Hopkins JM, Vittorio CC, Rook AH. CD8+ epidermotropic cytotoxic T-cell lymphoma with peripheral blood and central nervous system involvement. Arch Dermatol. 2008;144(8):1027–9.
65. Santucci M, Pimpinelli N, Massi D, et al. Cytotoxic/natural killer cell cutaneous lymphomas. Report of EORTC Cutaneous Lymphoma Task Force Workshop. Cancer. 2003;97(3):610–27.
66. Willemze R, Jaffe ES, Burg G, et al. WHO-EORTC classification for cutaneous lymphomas. Blood. 2005;105(10):3768–85.
67. Gonzalez CL, Medeiros LJ, Braziel RM, Jaffe ES. T-cell lymphoma involving subcutaneous tissue. A clinicopathologic entity commonly associated with hemophagocytic syndrome. Am J Surg Pathol. 1991;15(1):17–27.
68. Willemze R, Jansen PM, Cerroni L, et al. Subcutaneous panniculitis-like T-cell lymphoma: definition, classification, and prognostic factors: an EORTC Cutaneous Lymphoma Group Study of 83 cases. Blood. 2008;111(2):838–45.
69. Arnulf B, Copie-Bergman C, Delfau-Larue MH, et al. Nonhepatosplenic gammadelta T-cell lymphoma: a subset of cytotoxic lymphomas with mucosal or skin localization. Blood. 1998;91(5):1723–31.
70. Massone C, Chott A, Metze D, et al. Subcutaneous, blastic natural killer (NK), NK/T-cell, and other cytotoxic lymphomas of the skin: a morphologic, immunophenotypic, and molecular study of 50 patients. Am J Surg Pathol. 2004;28(6):719–35.
71. Toro JR, Beaty M, Sorbara L, et al. gamma delta T-cell lymphoma of the skin: a clinical, microscopic, and molecular study. Arch Dermatol. 2000;136(8):1024–32.
72. Jones D, Vega F, Sarris AH, Medeiros LJ. CD4-CD8-"Double-negative" cutaneous T-cell lymphomas share common histologic features and an aggressive clinical course. Am J Surg Pathol. 2002;26(2):225–31.
73. Tokura YJE, Sander CA. Cutaneous adult T-cell leukaemia/lymphoma. In: LeBoit PEBG, Weedon D, Sarasin A, editors. Pathology and genetics of skin tumors. Lyon: IARC; 2006. pp. 189–90.
74. Yagi H, Takigawa M, Hashizume H. Cutaneous type of adult T cell leukemia/lymphoma: a new entity among cutaneous lymphomas. J Dermatol. 2003;30(9):641–3.
75. Shimoyama M. Diagnostic criteria and classification of clinical subtypes of adult T-cell leukaemia-lymphoma. A report from the Lymphoma Study Group (1984–87). Br J Haematol. 1991;79(3):428–37.
76. Tsukasaki K, Hermine O, Bazarbachi A, et al. Definition, prognostic factors, treatment, and response criteria of adult T-cell leukemia-lymphoma: a proposal from an international consensus meeting. J Clin Oncol. 2009;27(3):453–9.
77. Chuang SS. Cutaneous non-MF T-cell and NK-cell lymphoproliferative disorders. In: MJ M, editor. Molecular diagnostics in dermatology and dermatopathology. New York: Humana Press; 2011. pp. 241–2.
78. Chan JKCQ-ML, Ferry JA, Peh SC. Extranodal NK/T-cell lymphoma, nasal-type. In: Swerdlow SHCE, Harris NL, et al. editor. WHO classification of tumours of haematopoietic and lymphoid tissues. Lyon: IARC; 2008. pp. 285–8.
79. Arber DA, Weiss LM, Albujar PF, Chen YY, Jaffe ES. Nasal lymphomas in Peru. High incidence of T-cell immunophenotype and Epstein-Barr virus infection. Am J Surg Pathol. 1993;17(4):392–9.
80. Chan JK. Natural killer cell neoplasms. Anat Pathol. 1998;3:77–145.
81. Au WY, Weisenburger DD, Intragumtornchai T, et al. Clinical differences between nasal and extranasal natural killer/T-cell lymphoma: a study of 136 cases from the International Peripheral T-Cell Lymphoma Project. Blood. 2009;113(17):3931–7.
82. Jaffe ES. Nasal and nasal-type T/NK cell lymphoma: a unique form of lymphoma associated with the Epstein-Barr virus. Histopathology. 1995;27(6):581–3.
83. Tsang WY, Chan JK, Yip TT, et al. In situ localization of Epstein-Barr virus encoded RNA in non-nasal/nasopharyngeal CD56-positive and CD56-negative T-cell lymphomas. Hum Pathol. 1994;25(8):758–65.

84.   Liao JB, Chuang SS, Chen HC, Tseng HH, Wang JS, Hsieh PP. Clinicopathologic analysis of cutaneous lymphoma in taiwan: a high frequency of extranodal natural killer/t-cell lymphoma, nasal type, with an extremely poor prognosis. Arch Pathol Lab Med. 2010;134(7):996–1002.
85.   Jaffe ES, Chan JK, Su IJ, et al. Report of the workshop on nasal and related extranodal angiocentric T/natural killer cell lymphomas. Definitions, differential diagnosis, and epidemiology. Am J Surg Pathol. 1996;20(1):103–11.
86.   Rodriguez J, Romaguera JE, Manning J, et al. Nasal-type T/NK lymphomas: a clinicopathologic study of 13 cases. Leuk Lymphoma. 2000;39(1–2):139–44.
87.   Gaal K, Sun NC, Hernandez AM, Arber DA. Sinonasal NK/T-cell lymphomas in the United States. Am J Surg Pathol. 2000;24(11):1511–7.
88.   Lin CW, Lee WH, Chang CL, Yang JY, Hsu SM. Restricted killer cell immunoglobulin-like receptor repertoire without T-cell receptor gamma rearrangement supports a true natural killer-cell lineage in a subset of sinonasal lymphomas. Am J Pathol. 2001;159(5):1671–9.
89.   Kohler S, Iwatsuki K, Jaffe ES, Chan JKC. Extranodal NK/T-cell lymphoma, nasal type. In: LeBoit PEBG, Weedon D, Sarasin A, editors Pathology and genetics of skin tumors. Lyon: IARC; 2006. pp. 191–2.
90.   Barrionuevo C, Anderson VM, Zevallos-Giampietri E, et al. Hydroa-like cutaneous T-cell lymphoma: a clinicopathologic and molecular genetic study of 16 pediatric cases from Peru. Appl Immunohistochem Mol Morphol. 2002;10(1):7–14.
91.   Iwatsuki K, Ohtsuka M, Akiba H, Kaneko F. Atypical hydroa vacciniforme in childhood: from a smoldering stage to Epstein-Barr virus-associated lymphoid malignancy. J Am Acad Dermatol. 1999;40(2 Pt 1):283–4.
92.   Iwatsuki K, Satoh M, Yamamoto T, et al. Pathogenic link between hydroa vacciniforme and Epstein-Barr virus-associated hematologic disorders. Arch Dermatol. 2006;142(5):587–95.
93.   Rodriguez-Pinilla SM, Barrionuevo C, Garcia J, et al. EBV-associated cutaneous NK/T-cell lymphoma: review of a series of 14 cases from peru in children and young adults. Am J Surg Pathol. 2010;34(12):1773–82.
94.   Magana M, Sangueza P, Gil-Beristain J, et al. Angiocentric cutaneous T-cell lymphoma of childhood (hydroa-like lymphoma): a distinctive type of cutaneous T-cell lymphoma. J Am Acad Dermatol. 1998;38(4):574–9.
95.   Yamamoto T, Tsuji K, Suzuki D, Morizane S, Iwatsuki K. A novel, noninvasive diagnostic probe for hydroa vacciniforme and related disorders: detection of latency-associated Epstein-Barr virus transcripts in the crusts. J Microbiol Methods. 2007;68(2):403–7.
96.   Zelger B, Sepp N, Weyrer K, Grunewald K. Syringotropic cutaneous T-cell lymphoma: a variant of mycosis fungoides? Br J Dermatol. 1994;130(6):765–9.
97.   Wood GS, Kamath NV, Guitart J, et al. Absence of Borrelia burgdorferi DNA in cutaneous B-cell lymphomas from the United States. J Cutan Pathol. 2001;28(10):502–7.
98.   Kempf W, Ralfkiaer E, Duncan L, Burg G, Willemze R, Swerdlow SH, Jaffe ES. Cutaneous marginal zone B-cell lymphoma. In: LeBoit PE, Burg G, Weedon D, Sarasin A, editors. Pathology and genetics of skin tumors. Lyon: IARC; 2006. pp. 194–5.
99.   Baldassano MF, Bailey EM, Ferry JA, Harris NL, Duncan LM. Cutaneous lymphoid hyperplasia and cutaneous marginal zone lymphoma: comparison of morphologic and immunophenotypic features. Am J Surg Pathol. 1999;23(1):88–96.
100. Gallardo F, Bellosillo B, Serrano S, Pujol RM. [Genotypic analysis in primary cutaneous lymphomas using the standardized BIOMED-2 polymerase chain reaction protocols]. Actas Dermosifiliogr. 2008;99(8):608–20.
101. Swerdlow SHCEHN, Jaffe ES, Pileri SA, Stein H, Thiele J, Vardiman JW. World health organization classification of tumors of hematopoietic and lymphoid tissues. Lyon: IARC; 2008.
102. Li C, Inagaki H, Kuo TT, Hu S, Okabe M, Eimoto T. Primary cutaneous marginal zone B-cell lymphoma: a molecular and clinicopathologic study of 24 asian cases. Am J Surg Pathol. 2003;27(8):1061–9.

103. Cerroni L, Arzberger E, Putz B, et al. Primary cutaneous follicle center cell lymphoma with follicular growth pattern. Blood. 2000;95(12):3922–8.

104. de Leval L, Ferry JA, Falini B, Shipp M, Harris NL. Expression of bcl-6 and CD10 in primary mediastinal large B-cell lymphoma: evidence for derivation from germinal center B cells? Am J Surg Pathol. 2001;25(10):1277–82.

105. Cerroni L, Volkenandt M, Rieger E, Soyer HP, Kerl H. bcl-2 protein expression and correlation with the interchromosomal 14;18 translocation in cutaneous lymphomas and pseudolymphomas. J Invest Dermatol. 1994;102(2):231–5.

106. Vergier B, Belaud-Rotureau MA, Benassy MN, et al. Neoplastic cells do not carry bcl2-JH rearrangements detected in a subset of primary cutaneous follicle center B-cell lymphomas. Am J Surg Pathol. 2004;28(6):748–55.

107. Dijkman R, Tensen CP, Jordanova ES, et al. Array-based comparative genomic hybridization analysis reveals recurrent chromosomal alterations and prognostic parameters in primary cutaneous large B-cell lymphoma. J Clin Oncol. 2006;24(2):296–305.

108. Hallermann C, Kaune KM, Siebert R, et al. Chromosomal aberration patterns differ in subtypes of primary cutaneous B cell lymphomas. J Invest Dermatol. 2004;122(6):1495–502.

109. Paulli M, Viglio A, Vivenza D, et al. Primary cutaneous large B-cell lymphoma of the leg: histogenetic analysis of a controversial clinicopathologic entity. Hum Pathol. 2002;33(9):937–43.

110. Bradford PT, Devesa SS, Anderson WF, Toro JR. Cutaneous lymphoma incidence patterns in the United States: a population-based study of 3884 cases. Blood. 2009;113(21):5064–73.

111. Lair G, Parant E, Tessier MH, Jumbou O, Dreno B. Primary cutaneous B-cell lymphomas of the lower limbs: a study of integrin expression in 11 cases. Acta Derm Venereol. 2000;80(5):367–9.

112. Vermeer MH, Geelen FA, van Haselen CW, et al. Primary cutaneous large B-cell lymphomas of the legs. A distinct type of cutaneous B-cell lymphoma with an intermediate prognosis. Dutch cutaneous lymphoma working group. Arch Dermatol. 1996;132(11):1304–8.

113. Senff NJ, Hoefnagel JJ, Jansen PM, et al. Reclassification of 300 primary cutaneous B-Cell lymphomas according to the new WHO-EORTC classification for cutaneous lymphomas: comparison with previous classifications and identification of prognostic markers. J Clin Oncol. 2007;25(12):1581–7.

114. Geelen FA, Vermeer MH, Meijer CJ, et al. bcl-2 protein expression in primary cutaneous large B-cell lymphoma is site-related. J Clin Oncol. 1998;16(6):2080–5.

115. Mao X, Lillington D, Child F, Russell-Jones R, Young B, Whittaker S. Comparative genomic hybridization analysis of primary cutaneous B-cell lymphomas: identification of common genomic alterations in disease pathogenesis. Genes Chromosomes Cancer. 2002;35(2):144–55.

116. Hoefnagel JJ, Dijkman R, Basso K, et al. Distinct types of primary cutaneous large B-cell lymphoma identified by gene expression profiling. Blood. 2005;105(9):3671–8.

117. Swerdlow SHCE, Harris NL, Jaffe ES, Pileri SA, Stein H, Thiele J, Vardiman JW. World Health Organization classification of tumors of hematopoietic and lymphoid tissues. Lyon: IARC; 2008.

118. Cho-Vega JH, Medeiros LJ, Prieto VG, Vega F. Leukemia cutis. Am J Clin Pathol. 2008;129(1):130–42.

119. Cronin DM, George TI, Sundram UN. An updated approach to the diagnosis of myeloid leukemia cutis. Am J Clin Pathol. 2009;132(1):101–10.

120. Hejmadi RK, Thompson D, Shah F, Naresh KN. Cutaneous presentation of aleukemic monoblastic leukemia cutis—a case report and review of literature with focus on immunohistochemistry. J Cutan Pathol. 2008;35 Suppl 1:46–9.

121. Sotiriou E, Manousari A, Apalla Z, Papagarifallou I, Ioannides D. Aleukaemic congenital leukaemia cutis: a critical primary sign of systemic disease. Acta Derm Venereol. 2011;91(2):203–4.

122. Deeb G, Baer MR, Gaile DP, et al. Genomic profiling of myeloid sarcoma by array comparative genomic hybridization. Genes Chromosomes Cancer. 2005;44(4):373–83.

123. Pileri SA, Ascani S, Cox MC, et al. Myeloid sarcoma: clinico-pathologic, phenotypic and cytogenetic analysis of 92 adult patients. Leukemia. 2007;21(2):340–50.
124. Wrede JE, Sundram U, Kohler S, Cherry AM, Arber DA, George TI. Fluorescence in situ hybridization investigation of cutaneous lesions in acute promyelocytic leukemia. Mod Pathol. 2005;18(12):1569–76.
125. Mao X, Lillington DM, Czepulkowski B, Young BD, Russell-Jones R, Whittaker S. A case of adult T-cell leukaemia/lymphoma characterized by multiplex-fluorescence in situ hybridization, comparative genomic hybridization, fluorescence in situ hybridization and cytogenetics. Br J Dermatol. 2001;145(1):117–22.
126. Murphy M. Leukemia cutis. In: Murphy MJ, editor. Molecular diagnostics in dermatology and dermatopathology. New York: Humana Press; 2011.
127. Scholl S, Luftner J, Mugge LO, Schmidt V, Fricke HJ, Hoffken K. Sustained expression of nucleophosmin (NPM1) mutation at late relapse presenting as isolated myeloid sarcoma in a patient with acute myeloid leukemia. Ann Hematol. 2007;86(10):763–5.
128. Sen F, Zhang XX, Prieto VG, Shea CR, Qumsiyeh MB. Increased incidence of trisomy 8 in acute myeloid leukemia with skin infiltration (leukemia cutis). Diagn Mol Pathol. 2000;9(4):190–4.
129. Douet-Guilbert N, Morel F, Bris MJ L, Sassolas B, Giroux JD, De Braekeleer M. Rearrangement of MLL in a patient with congenital acute monoblastic leukemia and granulocytic sarcoma associated with a t(1;11)(p36;q23) translocation. Leuk Lymphoma. 2005;46(1):143–6.
130. Byrd JC, Edenfield WJ, Shields DJ, Dawson NA. Extramedullary myeloid cell tumors in acute nonlymphocytic leukemia: a clinical review. J Clin Oncol. 1995;13(7):1800–16.
131. Watson KM, Mufti G, Salisbury JR, du Vivier AW, Creamer D. Spectrum of clinical presentation, treatment and prognosis in a series of eight patients with leukaemia cutis. Clin Exp Dermatol. 2006;31(2):218–21.
132. Benet C, Gomez A, Aguilar C, et al. Histologic and immunohistologic characterization of skin localization of myeloid disorders: a study of 173 cases. Am J Clin Pathol. 2011;135(2):278–90.
133. Pedersen J, Carganello J, van der Weyden MB. Exaggerated reaction to insect bites in patients with chronic lymphocytic leukemia. Clinical and histological findings. Pathology. 1990;22(3):141–3.
134. Bergman R. Pseudolymphoma and cutaneous lymphoma: facts and controversies. Clin Dermatol. 2010;28(5):568–74.
135. Gutermuth J, Audring H, Roseeuw D. Disseminated cutaneous B-cell lymphoma mimicking pseudolymphoma over a period of six years. Am J Dermatopathol. 2004;26(3):225–9.
136. Schiller PI, Flaig MJ, Puchta U, Kind P, Sander CA. Detection of clonal T cells in lichen planus. Arch Dermatol Res. 2000;292(11):568–9.
137. Boer A, Bresch M, Dayrit J, Falk TM. Erythema migrans: a reassessment of diagnostic criteria for early cutaneous manifestations of borreliosis with particular emphasis on clonality investigations. Br J Dermatol. 2007;156(6):1263–71.
138. Magro C, Crowson AN, Kovatich A, Burns F. Pityriasis lichenoides: a clonal T-cell lymphoproliferative disorder. Hum Pathol. 2002;33(8):788–95.
139. Arai E, Shimizu M, Tsuchida T, Izaki S, Ogawa F, Hirose T. Lymphomatoid keratosis: an epidermotropic type of cutaneous lymphoid hyperplasia: clinicopathological, immunohistochemical, and molecular biological study of 6 cases. Arch Dermatol. 2007;143(1):53–9.
140. Aram G, Rohwedder A, Nazeer T, Shoss R, Fisher A, Carlson JA. Varicella-zoster-virus folliculitis promoted clonal cutaneous lymphoid hyperplasia. Am J Dermatopathol. 2005;27(5):411–7.
141. Boer A, Tirumalae R, Bresch M, Falk TM. Pseudoclonality in cutaneous pseudolymphomas: a pitfall in interpretation of rearrangement studies. Br J Dermatol. 2008;159(2):394–402.

142. Conde-Taboada A, Roson E, Fernandez-Redondo V, Garcia-Doval I, De La TC, Cruces M. Lymphomatoid contact dermatitis induced by gold earrings. Contact Dermatitis. 2007;56(3):179–81.
143. Houck HE, Wirth FA, Kauffman CL. Lymphomatoid contact dermatitis caused by nickel. Am J Contact Dermat. 1997;8(3):175–6.
144. Evans AV, Banerjee P, McFadden JP, Calonje E. Lymphomatoid contact dermatitis to paratertyl-butyl phenol resin. Clin Exp Dermatol. 2003;28(3):272–3.
145. Ezzedine K, Rafii N, Heenen M. Lymphomatoid contact dermatitis to an exotic wood: a very harmful toilet seat. Contact Dermatitis. 2007;57(2):128–30.
146. Candiago E, Marocolo D, Manganoni MA, Leali C, Facchetti F. Nonlymphoid intraepidermal mononuclear cell collections (pseudo-Pautrier abscesses): a morphologic and immunophenotypical characterization. Am J Dermatopathol. 2000;22(1):1–6.
147. Burkert KL, Huhn K, Menezes DW, Murphy GF. Langerhans cell microgranulomas (pseudo-pautrier abscesses): morphologic diversity, diagnostic implications and pathogenetic mechanisms. J Cutan Pathol. 2002;29(9):511–6.
148. Wolff-Sneedorff A, Thomsen K, Secher L, Vejlsgaard GL. Gene rearrangement in positive patch tests. Exp Dermatol. 1995;4(5):322–6.
149. Simon M, Flaig MJ, Kind P, Sander CA, Kaudewitz P. Large plaque parapsoriasis: clinical and genotypic correlations. J Cutan Pathol. 2000;27(2):57–60.
150. Lazar AP, Caro WA, Roenigk HH Jr, Pinski KS. Parapsoriasis and mycosis fungoides: the Northwestern University experience, 1970 to 1985. J Am Acad Dermatol. 1989;21(5 Pt 1):919–23.
151. Kikuchi A, Naka W, Harada T, Sakuraoka K, Harada R, Nishikawa T. Parapsoriasis en plaques: its potential for progression to malignant lymphoma. J Am Acad Dermatol. 1993;29(3):419–22.
152. Burg G, Dummer R, Nestle FO, Doebbeling U, Haeffner A. Cutaneous lymphomas consist of a spectrum of nosologically different entities including mycosis fungoides and small plaque parapsoriasis. Arch Dermatol. 1996;132(5):567–72.
153. Vakeva L, Sarna S, Vaalasti A, Pukkala E, Kariniemi AL, Ranki A. A retrospective study of the probability of the evolution of parapsoriasis en plaques into mycosis fungoides. Acta Derm Venereol. 2005;85(4):318–23.
154. Bowers S, Warshaw EM. Pityriasis lichenoides and its subtypes. J Am Acad Dermatol. 2006;55(4):557–72. quiz 573–556.
155. Dereure O, Levi E, Kadin ME. T-Cell clonality in pityriasis lichenoides et varioliformis acuta: a heteroduplex analysis of 20 cases. Arch Dermatol. 2000;136(12):1483–6.
156. Shieh S, Mikkola DL, Wood GS. Differentiation and clonality of lesional lymphocytes in pityriasis lichenoides chronica. Arch Dermatol. 2001;137(3):305–8.
157. Smoller BR, Kamel OW. Pigmented purpuric eruptions: immunopathologic studies supportive of a common immunophenotype. J Cutan Pathol. 1991;18(6):423–7.
158. Magro CM, Schaefer JT, Crowson AN, Li J, Morrison C. Pigmented purpuric dermatosis: classification by phenotypic and molecular profiles. Am J Clin Pathol. 2007;128(2):218–29.
159. Boyd AS, Vnencak-Jones CL. T-cell clonality in lichenoid purpura: a clinical and molecular evaluation of seven patients. Histopathology. 2003;43(3):302–3.
160. Toro JR, Sander CA, LeBoit PE. Persistent pigmented purpuric dermatitis and mycosis fungoides: simulant, precursor, or both? A study by light microscopy and molecular methods. Am J Dermatopathol. 1997;19(2):108–18.
161. Fink-Puches R, Wolf P, Kerl H, Cerroni L. Lichen aureus: clinicopathologic features, natural history, and relationship to mycosis fungoides. Arch Dermatol. 2008;144(9):1169–73.
162. Requena L, Sanchez Yus E Panniculitis. Part II. Mostly lobular panniculitis. J Am Acad Dermatol. 2001;45(3):325–61. quiz 362–324.
163. Massone C, Kodama K, Salmhofer W, et al. Lupus erythematosus panniculitis (lupus profundus): clinical, histopathological, and molecular analysis of nine cases. J Cutan Pathol. 2005;32(6):396–404.

164. Park HS, Choi JW, Kim BK, Cho KH. Lupus erythematosus panniculitis: clinicopathological, immunophenotypic, and molecular studies. Am J Dermatopathol. 2010;32(1):24–30.
165. Magro CM, Crowson AN, Kovatich AJ, Burns F. Lupus profundus, indeterminate lymphocytic lobular panniculitis and subcutaneous T-cell lymphoma: a spectrum of subcuticular T-cell lymphoid dyscrasia. J Cutan Pathol. 2001;28(5):235–47.
166. Magro CM, Schaefer JT, Morrison C, Porcu P. Atypical lymphocytic lobular panniculitis: a clonal subcutaneous T-cell dyscrasia. J Cutan Pathol. 2008;35(10):947–54.
167. Petit T, Cribier B, Bagot M, Wechsler J. Inflammatory vitiligo-like macules that simulate hypopigmented mycosis fungoides. Eur J Dermatol. 2003;13(4):410–2.
168. Horn TD, Abanmi A. Analysis of the lymphocytic infiltrate in a case of vitiligo. Am J Dermatopathol. 1997;19(4):400–2.
169. Werner B, Massone C, Kerl H, Cerroni L. Large CD30-positive cells in benign, atypical lymphoid infiltrates of the skin. J Cutan Pathol. 2008;35(12):1100–7.
170. Fukamachi S, Sugita K, Sawada Y, Bito T, Nakamura M, Tokura Y. Drug-induced CD30+ T cell pseudolymphoma. Eur J Dermatol. 2009;19(3):292–4.
171. Colli C, Leinweber B, Mullegger R, Chott A, Kerl H, Cerroni L. Borrelia burgdorferi-associated lymphocytoma cutis: clinicopathologic, immunophenotypic, and molecular study of 106 cases. J Cutan Pathol. 2004;31(3):232–40.
172. Bergman R, Khamaysi K, Khamaysi Z, Ben Arie Y. A study of histologic and immunophenotypical staining patterns in cutaneous lymphoid hyperplasia. J Am Acad Dermatol. 65(1):112–24.
173. Ceballos KM, Gascoyne RD, Martinka M, Trotter MJ. Heavy multinodular cutaneous lymphoid infiltrates: clinicopathologic features and B-cell clonality. J Cutan Pathol. 2002;29(3):159–67.
174. Jung J, Levin EC, Jarrett R, Lu D, Mann C. Lymphomatoid drug reaction to ustekinumab. Arch Dermatol. 147(8):992–3.
175. Leo AM, Ermolovich T. Lymphomatoid papulosis while on efalizumab. J Am Acad Dermatol. 2009;61(3):540–1.
176. Magro CM, Crowson AN, Kovatich AJ, Burns F. Drug-induced reversible lymphoid dyscrasia: a clonal lymphomatoid dermatitis of memory and activated T cells. Hum Pathol. 2003;34(2):119–29.

Chapter 3
Molecular Testing in Cutaneous Mesenchymal Tumors

Wei-Lien Wang and Alexander J. Lazar

Introduction

Mesenchymal tumors can be difficult to diagnose, with those manifesting in the skin presenting unique challenges. Part of the difficultly comes from the rarity of these tumors ($< 1\,\%$ of all malignancies overall), in comparison to epithelial and melanocytic tumors. In addition, there are over 50 subtypes of mesenchymal tumors, each with a range of appearances that can histologically overlap with each other, including some benign and malignant entities [1]. Even the same tumor can have a wide range of histological, immunohistochemical, and clinical presentations. For example, mesenchymal tumors normally seen in bone or deep soft tissue can sometimes unexpectedly be present in the skin, either as a primary or metastasis [2–4].

Fortunately, a growing number of mesenchymal tumors have been discovered to harbor recurrent genetic aberrations (see Table 3.1). These alterations are not only important to tumorigenesis, but they can be used diagnostically. Mesenchymal tumors can be divided into two groups: those with relatively simple karyotypes with translocations and gene mutations and those with complex karyotypes, some of which also harbor gene amplification [5, 6]. Approximately, half of the mesenchymal tumors have recurrent translocations where two genes are fused together to create a new fusion or chimeric oncogene. Ewing sarcoma is a classic example where in the majority of the cases, there is a translocation involving the 5′ end promoter region of *EWSR1* located on 22q12 and the 3′ end on *FLI1* on 11q24 [7]. Gene mutation is another theme encountered in mesenchymal tumors. Constitutive activation of a proto-oncogene is most common, but loss of function in tumor suppressor genes is also seen, such as loss of the *SMARCB1* (*INI1*) gene in epithelioid sarcoma

W.-L. Wang (✉)
Department of Pathology, The University of Texas: MD Anderson
Cancer Center, 1515 Holcombe Blvd, Unit 85, Houston, TX 77030, USA
e-mail: wlwang@mdanderson.org

A. J. Lazar
Department of Pathology, The University of Texas: MD Anderson Cancer Center,
Houston, TX 77030, USA

© Springer Science+Business Media New York 2015
V. G. Prieto (ed.), *Precision Molecular Pathology of Dermatologic Diseases,*
Molecular Pathology Library 9, DOI 10.1007/978-1-4939-2861-3_3

Table 3.1 Selected mesenchymal tumors and their recurrent molecular alterations

Tumor type	Translocation/chromosome involved	Genes involved
Alveolar rhabdomyosarcoma	t(2;13))(q35;q14) t(1;13)(p36;q14) t(X;2)(q13;q35)	*PAX3-FKHR* *PAX7-FKHR* *PAX3-AFX*
Alveolar soft-part sarcoma	der(17)t(X;17)(p11;q25)	*ASPL-TFE3*
Angiomatoid fibrous histiocytoma	t(12;22)(q13;q12) t(2;22)(q33;q12) t(12;16)(q13;p11)	*EWSR1-ATF1* *EWSR1-CREB1* *FUS-ATF1*
Chondroid lipoma	t(11;16)(q13;p13)	*CLLorf95-MKL2*
Clear-cell sarcoma	t(12;22)(q13;q12) t(2;22)(q33;q12)	*EWSR1-AFT1* *EWSR1-CREB1*
Congenital/infantile fibrosarcoma	t(12;15)(p13;q25)	*ETV6-NTRK3*
Dermatofibrosarcoma protuberans (DFSP)	t(17;22)(q21;q13)	*COLIA1-PDGFB*
Desmoid fibromatosis	3p21 5q22	*CTNNB1* (sporadic) *APC* (FAP related)
Desmoplastic small round cell tumor	t(11;22)(p13;q12)	*EWSR1-WT1*
Epithelioid hemangioendothelioma	t(1;3)(p36;q25) t(11;21)(q22;q22)	*WWTR1-CAMTA1* *YAP1-TFE3*
Epithelioid sarcoma	22q11.23	*SMARCB1*
Ewing sarcoma: PNET	t(11;12)(q24;q12) t(21;22)(q22;q12) t(7;22)(p22;q12) t(2;22)(q33;q12) t(17;22)(q12;q12) inv(22)(q12;q12) t(16;21)(p11;q22)	*EWSR1-FLI1* *EWSR1-ERG* *EWSR1-ETV1* *EWSR1-FEV* *EWSR1-E1AF* *EWSR1-ZSG* *FUS-ERG*
"Ewing-like" tumors	t(4;19)(q35;q13) inv(X)(p11.4;p11.22)	*CIC-DUX4* *BCOR-CCNB3*
Extraskeletal myxoid chondrosarcoma	t(9;22)(q22;q12) t(9;17)(q22;q11) t(9;15)(q22;q21) t(3;9)(q11;q22)	*EWSR1-NR4A3* *TAF2N-NR4A3* *TCF12-NR4A3* *TFG-NR4A3*
Gastrointestinal stromal tumor	4q12 4q12	*KIT PDGFRFA*
Inflammatory myofibroblastic tumor	t(1;2)(q22;p23) t(2;19)(p23;p13) t(2;17)(p23;q23) t(2;2)(p23;q13) t(2;11)(p23;p15) inv(2)(p23;q35)	*TPM3-ALK* *TPM4-ALK* *CLTC-ALK* *RANB2-ALK* *CARS-ALK* *ATIC-ALK*
Lipoblastoma	8q11-13	*PLAG1, HMGA2* with various partners
Lipoma	12q13~15, 13q, 6p21~23	*HMGA2* with various partners (*LPP, CXCR7, EBF1, NFIB, LHFP*), subset of tumors
Low-grade fibromyxoid sarcoma	t(7;16)(q33;p11) t(11;16)(p11;p11)	*FUS-CREB3L2* *FUS-CREB3L1*

Table 3.1 (continued)

Tumor type	Translocation/chromosome involved	Genes involved
Mesenchymal chondrosarcoma	t(8;8)(q13;q21)	*HEY1-NCOA2*
Myoepithelial tumor of soft tissue	t(6;22)(p21;q12) t(19;22)(q13;q12) t(1;22)(q23;q12) t(1;16)(p34;p11) t(1;22)(p34;q12) 8q12 rearrangements	*EWSR1-POU5F1* *EWSR1-ZNF444* *EWSR1-PBX1* *FUS-KLF17* *EWSR1-KLF17* *PLAG1*
Myxoid/round-cell liposarcoma	t(12;16)(q13;p11) t(12;22)(q13;q12)	*FUS-DDIT3(TLS-CHOP)* *EWSR1-DDIT3(EWSR1-CHOP)*
Myxoinflammatory fibroblastic sarcoma/hemosiderotic fibrolipomatous tumor	t(1;10)(p22;q24) 3p11 ~ 12(ring chromosome)	*TGFBR3~MGEA5,* Amplification of *VGLL3, CHMP2B*
Nodular fasciitis	t(17;22)(p13;q13)	*MYH9-USP6*
Pseudomyogenic hemangioendothelioma	t(7;19)(q22;q13)	*SERPINE1-FOSB*
Sclerosing epithelioid fibrosarcoma	t(7;16)(p22;q24)	*FUS-CREB3L2*
Soft tissue angiofibroma	t(5;18)(p15;q13)	*AHRR-NCOA2*
Solitary fibrous tumor	inv(12)(q13;q13)	*NAB2-STAT6*
Synovial sarcoma	t(X;18)(p11;q11)	*SS18-SSX1, SSX2, SSX4*
Tenosynovial giant cell tumor/pigmented villonodular synovitis	t(1;2)(p13;q37)	*COL6A3-CSF*
Well differentiated liposarcoma/ALT/dedifferentiated liposarcoma	12q13 ~ 15(ring chromosomes, giant marker chromosomes)	Amplification of *MDM2, CDK4, HMGA2, GLI, SAS,* others

[8, 9]. An example of constitutive activation is gastrointestinal stromal tumor which can have various mutations (in frame deletions, insertions and point mutations) in the tyrosine kinase receptor genes, *KIT*, and/or *PDGFRA* [6, 10, 11]. These mutations result in constitutive activation of these receptors which also makes some of these tumors amendable to treatment by tyrosine kinase inhibitors, depending on the mutation type [10]. Another example of a tumor with an activating gene mutation is desmoid fibromatosis. These tumors have point mutations in *CTNNB1*, the gene that encodes for the protein β-catenin. This mutation prevents the breakdown of beta catenin and results in its nuclear accumulation which can be detected by immunohistochemistry study [12]. Finally, there is a subset of mesenchymal tumors that have complex karyotypes. Some of these have no known recurrent alteration, such as undifferentiated pleomorphic sarcoma. These tumors can have loss of function alterations in *TP53* and *Rb*, but such alterations are common in many types of neoplasia, both mesenchymal and non-mesenchymal and thus their diagnostic use is

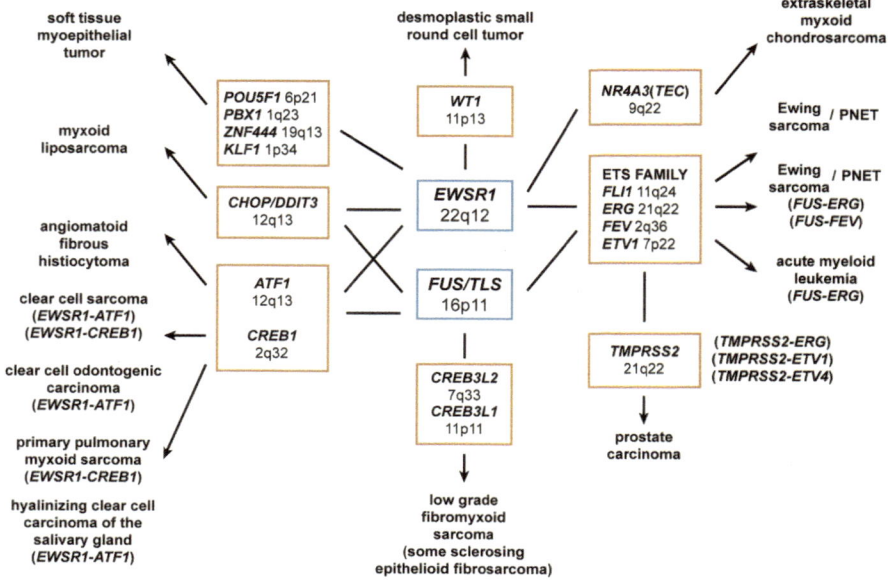

Fig. 3.1 Multiple mesenchymal tumors can share rearrangements in the same gene and even identical fusion transcripts.

limited [5]. Other tumors with complex karyotypes have gene amplification where portions or intervals of a chromosome and their corresponding genes are amplified. An example of this is atypical lipomatous tumor/well-differentiated liposarcoma/dedifferentiated liposarcoma, which have supernumerary ring and giant chromosomes with amplification of the 12q13~15 region, including the genes, *CDK4* and *MDM2* [13].

Previously, particular chromosomal rearrangements were considered to be specific to a particular mesenchymal tumor. However, this concept has evolved over several years as it is now understood that multiple tumors can have identical rearrangements (see Fig. 3.1). Chimeric genes involving *EWSR1* or *FUS* demonstrate this point well. Both genes are prominent players with many tumors and in some instances seem to even be used interchangeable as oncogenic promoters by the same tumor [1, 5, 14, 15]. These same genes are also not exclusive to mesenchymal tumors but can be seen in tumors of other lineages, including leukemia and carcinoma. Not only can mesenchymal tumors involve the same gene but they can share the exact same translocations. The most commonly cited example of this is clear cell sarcoma and angiomatoid fibrous histiocytoma [16–20]. Both have translocations involving *EWSR1* (22q12) and *ATF1* (12q13) and/or *CREB1* (2q34), yet are phenotypically divergent. Clear cell sarcoma is an aggressive tumor with melanocytic differentiation, while angiomatoid fibrous histiocytoma is an indolent tumor with uncertain differentiation. Although important to tumoriogenesis, other factors are clearly involved for phenotypic development in these tumors besides the single translocation. Interestingly, some of these same translocations can be seen in another recently described sarcoma, primary pulmonary myxoid sarcoma, and also carcinomas, such as hyalinizing clear cell carcinoma of the salivary gland and clear cell odontogenic carcinoma [21–24]. Even amplification involving the same regions can be seen in very different tumors, such as well-differentiated liposarcoma and well-differenti-ated osteosarcoma, both of which have amplification of 12q13~15 [25]. This phe-nomenon of shared genes, translocations and genetic alterations also highlights the importance of correlating molecular results with histology, immunohistochemical, and clinical findings to ensure that the correct interpretation is made. With advances in next generation sequencing techniques, additional discoveries continue to further our understanding of these rare tumors which can be useful diagnostically, as well as offer a potential therapeutic target.

Molecular Techniques

Multiple ancillary molecular techniques are available to pathologists. Each tech-nique carries unique strengths and weaknesses. It is important to be familiar with these features as they may influence which assay is best for a given situation. Cyto-genetic karyotyping has been long considered the gold standard in detecting genetic aberrations, and has given rise to many of the discoveries today [6]. Fresh tissue is obtained so that tumor cells can be grown and then processed so that metaphase chromosomes can be examined (Fig. 3.2). Fluorescently labeled probes can some-times be applied to identify the chromosomes (also known as spectral karyotyping) or to detect rearrangements of specific genes (see below for fluorescence in situ hybridization). An advantage of this technique is that it requires no prior knowledge of the genetic aberration and thus can detect a wide range of translocations and chromosomal abnormalities. This is particularly useful when dealing with difficult-to-diagnose mesenchymal tumors and where the identification of an unexpected translocation may provide clues to further classification, such as unusual histologi-cal or immunohistochemical variants. However, this technique requires fresh tis-sue, which is not always available. Lengthy processing time, expert technical staff, complex interpretation, bacterial contamination or normal tissue overgrowth, and associated costs can be negative issues. Finally, the technique cannot detect small mutations and translocations where the genes are in close proximity to each other (also known as cryptic translocations.) As a result, conventional karyotyping has largely given way to faster molecular techniques which have been optimized for formalin-fixed paraffin-embedded (FFPE) tissue.

One of the most widely used molecular technique for detecting translocations is fluorescence in situ hybridization (FISH) because of its robustness and broad util-ity in frozen, FFPE and cytological tissues. In this technique, fluorescently labelled DNA probes are applied to unstained slides. Interphase nuclei are examined under fluorescence microscope [6]. The most commonly available FISH assays are break-

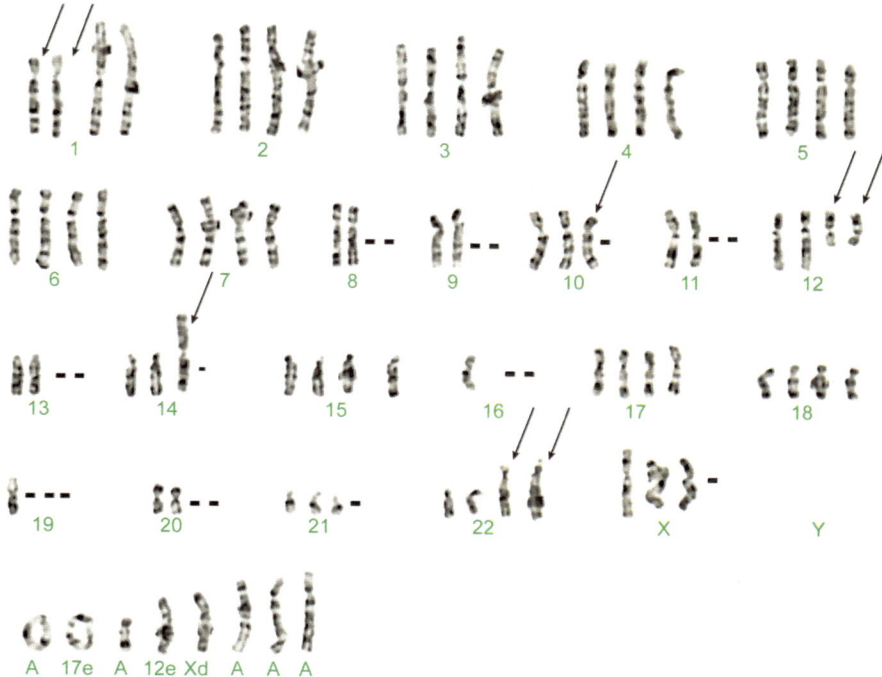

Fig. 3.2 Karyotype of a case of clear cell sarcoma showing a characteristic translocation involving chromosomes 12 and 22.

apart assays. In break-apart assays, two DNA probes flank a single gene of interest (Fig. 3.3). For example, in the *EWSR1* break-apart assay, two DNA probes flank the *EWSR1*, one in the 5′ end labeled with a probe which will fluorescence orange and one in the 3′ end with a probe which will fluorescence green. In tumors where *EWSR1* is not rearranged, both orange- and green-labeled probes co-localize to produce a yellow signal because of their spectral overlap when in close proximity to each other. In contrast, tumors where *EWSR1* is rearranged will have split signals, one separate orange and one separate green signal. FISH assays with fusion probes will also have two DNA probes but one for every involved genes. For example, in a fusion FISH assay for Ewing sarcoma, one probe will be bound to the 5′ *EWSR1* end, while a second probe will be bound to the 3′ end of *FLI1*. In contrast to the break-apart assays, tumors without rearrangement will have split signals, while tumors with rearrangements will have both probes next to other, co-localizing into a single yellow signal. In practice, break-apart FISH is a much more common approach as it covers a wider range of events with a single set of probes. The strengths of using FISH include its robustness in multiple tissues; most notably in FFPE tissue, the most commonly available tissue. Because it is in situ, the test is interpreted within tumor nuclei, something not possible in polymerase chain reactions (PCRs; see below). Furthermore, it is much faster than karyotyping as it does not require

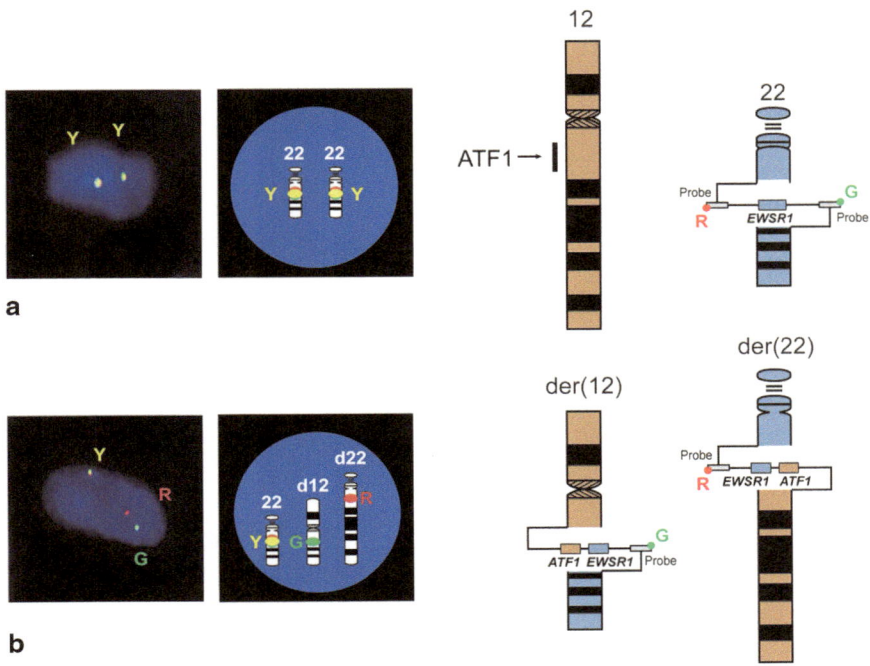

Fig. 3.3 Break-apart fluorescence in situ hybridization (FISH) assay for *EWSR1*. Example shown is of clear cell sarcoma. **a**. In tumors which are negative for rearrangement, DNA probes flanking *EWSR1* (one *green* and one *red*) co-localize to produce a *yellow* signal. **b**. In tumors with *EWSR1* rearrangement, the signals are split.

time for cells to grow. One disadvantage of FISH is that prior knowledge of a gene to target is needed. Furthermore, most commercially available FISH are break-apart assays that do not provide information on partner. Therefore, it cannot be used to differentiate similar appearing entities which have the same gene involved. For example, Ewing sarcoma and desmoplastic small round cell sarcoma are both small round cell tumors and both have rearrangements involving *EWSR1*, though with different partners. Break-apart FISH for *EWSR1* cannot be used to distinguish between these two entities. Another disadvantage is that multiplexing (ability to screen multiple gene aberrations at the same time) is limited as each assay typically requires an unstained slide, and is compounded by the fact that only a few DNA probes are commercially available.

Polymerase chain reaction (PCR) and reverse transcriptase-polymerase chain reaction (RT-PCR) have become common ancillary diagnostic assays for mesenchymal tumors [6]. DNA primers flank the gene or fusion gene of interest, are amplified several fold and sequenced to determine if mutation is present or not (Fig. 3.4). In RT-PCR, fusion transcript RNA is converted to DNA (cDNA) first. The major advantage of this technique is that it detects a specific gene fusion, providing information on both gene partners. This is important when knowledge of partner genes is

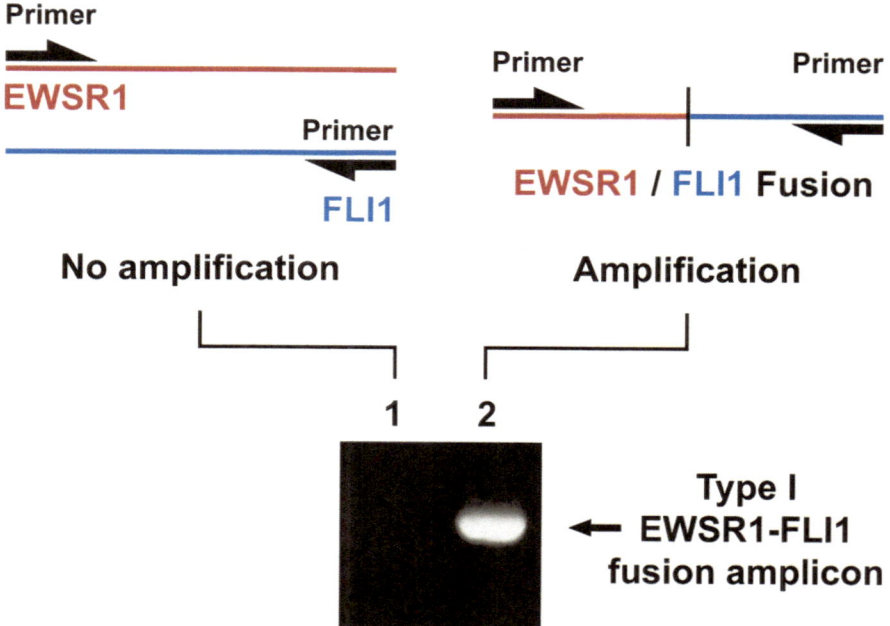

Fig. 3.4 PCR primers flank DNA or cDNA of interest (example shown is *EWSR1-FLI1* cDNA). Samples containing a fusion transcript will result in a band on electrophoresis which can be sequenced for confirmation.

needed to differentiate between two similar appearing tumors. As mentioned earlier, break-apart FISH for *EWSR1* would not be useful to distinguish between Ewing sarcoma and desmoplastic small round cell tumor. However, RT-PCR would be able to discriminate between Ewing sarcoma (*EWSR1-FLI1* or *EWSR1-ERG*) and desmoplastic small round cell tumor (*EWSR1-WT1*), because it can specify fusion partners. Also, RNA extracted from unstained slides can be used to do multiple reactions. The major disadvantage of this technique is that it is not as robust as FISH. RNA is susceptible to degradation particularly in older FFPE blocks and decalcification. In addition, the majority of laboratories have assays which only detect the most common fusion transcript types and variants. A fusion transcript type is created between variations in breakpoints between the same genes, each of which is designated numerically as a type. For example, in Ewing sarcoma, there are multiple *EWSR1-FLI1* fusion types, with types I and II being most common. A fusion transcript variant is created with different genes. In Ewing sarcoma, *EWSR1* is most commonly paired with *FLI1*; however, it can also be paired with *ERG*, *FTV1*, and *FEV* among others to yield other variants. Therefore, it is possible that a less common variant or type is missed because the assay is not designed to detect them. One particular problematic tumor is dermatofibrosarcoma protuberans (DFSP) because it has multiple types due to substantial variation in break points within *COL1A1* which comprise more than 50 exons. Therefore, multiple primers are needed to

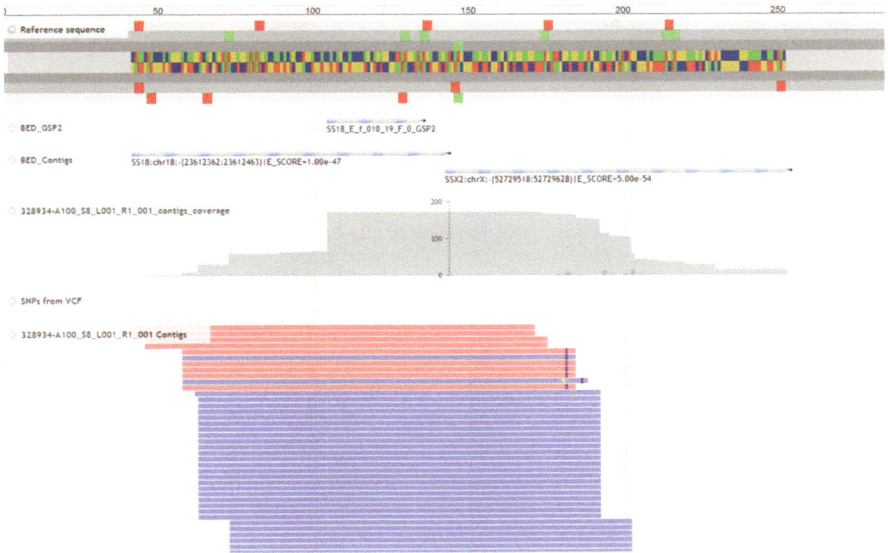

Fig. 3.5 While still evolving in both technique and bioinformatics interpretation, next generation sequencing approaches using semi-anchored amplification techniques are beginning to be employed in the clinical setting.

cover these many types [26]. Similar to FISH, commercial laboratories only offer a selected few RT-PCR assays. Finally, lack of in situ testing, raises the possibility that contamination can occur. Therefore, it is important to be confident that the laboratory chosen for such studies has solid protocols and impeccable procedures.

An exciting development in molecular diagnostics is the increasing utilization of next generation sequencing techniques. While global RNA sequencing (RNA-seq) is not ready for broad clinical application, semi-anchored approaches are being explored where primers specific for a common known gene is used with opposing nonspecific primers to theoretically identify any partner gene (Fig. 3.5). The bioinformatics for interpreting fusions is rapidly evolving and this is a growth area in molecular testing for translocations. Next generation sequencing can also be used to examine for broad panels of genes for point mutations, insertions, and deletions (and increasingly copy number alterations). These approaches have limited applications in sarcoma as the genomic properties of most sarcomas are poorly examined, but this is rapidly changing as new genomic analyses of sarcomas are being published regularly.

As in any assay, pre-analytical variables are important to consider prior to ordering a molecular diagnostic test. Such factors can explain a failed test or unexpected false negative. As alluded to earlier, RT-PCR assays are more sensitive to conditions, such as older tissue blocks, fixation (including over fixation), or decalcification as RNA is susceptible to being degraded in those conditions. Although these factors can also decrease its effectiveness as well, FISH which is DNA based is more robust. Hemorrhage and pigment can be problematic for both assays; these can inhibit polymerase enzymes causing the PCR assay to fail or result in auto-fluorescence in FISH making interpretation difficult. Sclerotic tissue and myxoid stroma can prevent FISH probes from penetrating into tumor nuclei or successful extraction of RNA. An abundance of normal tissue can be a cause for a false negative result. Therefore, it is important to enrich for tumor nuclei by circling an area of interest for FISH or macrodissection for extraction assays, such as RT-PCR as well as to avoid the above described problematic areas as much as possible.

Diagnostic Utility

In most situations, mesenchymal tumors can be diagnosed without molecular testing. However, molecular testing is very useful in certain situations including (1) additional support and reassurance in small biopsies, (2) unusual histological or immunohistochemical variants, (3) situations with unusual clinical presentation, and (4) evaluation for targeted therapy (sometimes required for a patient to qualify for clinical trial). Selected examples of common problematic situations with cutaneous mesenchymal tumors are discussed in detail below.

Clear Cell Sarcoma

Clear cell sarcoma is a high-grade sarcoma with melanocytic differentiation, which can be at times difficult to distinguish from melanoma that is metastatic or of unknown primary [1]. These tumors share histological features with enlarge nuclei, prominent nucleoli, amphophilic cytoplasm, and even melanosomes. Immunohistochemically, these tumors are also similar. Both are reactive for S-100 protein with those in the extremities expressing melanocytic markers diffusely, such as HMB45 and Mart-1. Clear cell sarcoma occurs in deep soft tissue, involving tendons and deep connective tissue of the extremities in young adults, and this can be helpful in favoring one over the other. However, melanoma (metastatic or of unknown primary) can also present in deep tissues; alternatively, clear cell sarcoma can involve the skin and dermis [4]. Given this overlap, molecular testing is useful to distinguish these two entities; either FISH testing for *EWSR1* rearrangement or RT-PCR for *EWSR1-ATF1* and *EWSR1-CREB1* fusion transcripts [18, 20, 27]. While *EWSR1-CREB1* fusion was initially thought to be exclusive to clear cell sarcoma-like tumor of the gastrointestinal tract (so called due to some differences in morphology and often lacking of HMB45 labeling), recent examples including cutaneous tumors, have also been found to harbor *EWSR1-CREB1* fusion transcripts [4, 18]. It is now understood that both transcript variants can be found in either location. Knowledge of what fusion transcript variants an assay covers is important as some laboratories may only test for one.

Dermatofibrosarcoma Protuberans

Dermatofibrosarcoma protuberans (DFSP) is a locally aggressive cutaneous tumor. Classically, these tumors are composed of CD34 positive short spindle cells arranged in a prominent storiform pattern involving the dermis and infiltrating into the subcutis and enveloping adipocytes. The infiltrative nature leads to a propensity for local recurrence and necessitates attention to ensure complete excision. Most cases are easily recognized by morphology and CD34 labeling [1]. However, diagnostic problems can arise with unusual morphological variants. Plaque-like atrophic variants with more elongated spindle fibrous cells and those with prominent myxoid stroma can complicate recognition, particularly on small and/or superficial biopsies [28, 29]. Rarely, these tumors can present predominantly in the subcutaneous soft tissue and be excised as a soft tissue mass without the dermal component. Finally, there can also be unusual morphological variants to fibrosarcomatous transformation. Fibrosarcomatous transformation heralds an increased risk of recurrence and, uncommon but documented (about 15 % risk), risk of metastasis over conventional DFSP. Fibrosarcomatous transformation is characterized by a sharp demarcation from the conventional areas with increased cellularity and mitotic activity, and monotonous spindled cells arranged in a fascicular to herringbone architecture [1, 30]. Partial or complete loss of CD34 can complicate recognition and the histological features can overlap with synovial sarcoma and malignant peripheral nerve sheath tumor. In addition, very unusual bizarre variants, including those with pleomorphic (mimicking an undifferentiated pleomorphic sarcoma), primitive small and giant cells (mimicking a giant cell tumor) can occur [31]. The diagnosis can be more challenging in cases where the fibrosarcomatous component obscures or obliterates the conventional component, or where a prior history of DFSP is not elicited with a fibrosarcomatous local or distant (such as lung) recurrence.

Fortunately, the majority of these tumors have rearrangements involving *COL1A1* on 17q21 and *PDGFB* on 22q13 [26]. As noted above, while the breakpoint consistently involves intron 1 (non-coding DNA) prior to exon 2 (coding DNA) of *PDGFB*, there are many breakpoints which span the 51 introns of *COL1A1*. As a result, multiple primers are required to cover as many fusion types and may be a cause for a false negative result. FISH also can be performed to look for *PDGFB* rearrangement, but the unusual nature of the rearrangement to create copy number alternations in the probed regions makes this procedure more challenging as well.

Molecular testing can be equally important in ruling out the diagnosis of DFSP when dealing with unusual cutaneous fibrohistiocytic lesions. Prior studies have described fibrohistiocytic lesions, which seem to have features of both dermatofibroma and dermatofibrosarcoma [32]. These lesions can even have a focally infiltrative growth pattern and significant CD34 and Factor 13a reactivity. Benign plaque-like dermal fibromas are also CD34 positive and can also be mistaken for DFSP [33]. The absence of rearrangement can provide reassurance in excluding the diagnosis and indicate a tumor will not necessarily behave the same as DFSP. This is also important as the juxtaposition of the *COL1A1* promoter with *PDGFB* in DFSP makes them amendable to tyrosine kinase inhibitors. This can be useful in reducing the tumor size in particularly sensitive areas (such as head and neck) and to increase the chance of a successful resection. Demonstration of the fusion may also provide a therapeutic option to patients with metastatic disease. Other tumors without this translocation would not be expected to respond similarly to this therapy.

Post-radiation Angiosarcoma

The distinction between atypical vascular tumors in post-radiated breast and post-radiation angiosarcoma can be challenging sometimes, particularly in small biopsies, and/or where clinical history is not well documented [34, 35]. Most post-radiation angiosarcomas are dermally located and aggressive, but can extend into the subcutis as well [1]. Occasionally, they can have very well-differentiated areas which makes them difficult to distinguish from other less aggressive vascular tumors, particularly on small biopsies. Atypical vascular lesions are small vascular proliferations with mild to moderate atypia but are concerning due to irregular vasoformative growth pattern and their occurrence in the prior radiation therapy field [34]. The small and well-circumscribed nature of these lesions is characteristic and thus a well-documented clinical examination is also very helpful in this setting.

Recently, c-myc (8q24) amplification has been demonstrated to be characteristic finding in the majority of post-radiation angiosarcomas while being absent in atypical vascular lesions [36, 37]. This copy number increase can be detected using FISH, with probes to the chromosome 8 centromere and to c-myc. Because c-myc amplification also results in MYC protein expression, MYC immunohistochemical study can also be a useful ancillary test.

Pseudomyogenic Hemangioendothelioma

Another rare vascular tumor that can involve the skin is pseudomyogenic hemangioendothelioma (also known as epithelioid sarcoma-like hemangioendothelioma). These tumors are composed of spindled cells with abundant eosinophilic cytoplasm and an inflammatory infiltrate. The tumor cells are reactive for both keratins and vascular markers (Erg, Fli1 and CD31) [1, 38, 39]. Histologically, these tumors can be mistaken for a smooth muscle tumor or epithelioid sarcoma. Recently, these tumors have been discovered to have a recurrent translocation involving SERPINE1 on 7q11 and FOSB on 19q13 [40]. Multiplex assays are developing to help detect and aid in the diagnosis in this rare tumor. FISH assays have also been described.

Myoepithelial Tumors of Soft Tissue

Cutaneous myoepithelial tumors are rare neoplasms that exhibit phenotypic features of both epithelial and mesenchymal tumors [1]. These tumors can have a wide range of morphological and immunohistochemical features making them challenging to diagnose. In contrast to their salivary gland counterparts, a subset of myoepithelial tumors of soft tissue have rearrangements involving *EWSR1* (22q12) or occasionally *FUS* (7p16) [41–43]. Multiple fusion partners have been described including *POU5F1* (8p21), *PBX-1* (1q23), and *ZNF44* (19q13); each fusion variant is reported to have some distinctive histologic finding, but more study is needed. *EWSR1* break-apart FISH assay can be helpful in diagnosing some of these tumors. Some tumors negative for *EWSR1/FUS* alterations have been found to have *PLAG1* rearrangements and ductal differentiation [44]. Multiplex fusion assays are currently being validated to detect multiple fusion partners. An important morphologic differential diagnosis is extraskeletal myxoid chondrosarcoma; a subset of these show *EWSR1* rearrangement as well [45]. (See Fig. 3.1) These are usually deeper soft tissue tumors and lack the immunohistochemical features characteristic of myoepithelial tumors.

Superficial Atypical Lipomatous Tumor

Most atypical lipomatous tumors/well-differentiated liposarcomas occur deep in the soft tissue. However, they can rarely have dermal presentations potentially resulting in diagnostic puzzlement [46–48]. Similar to their deeper counterparts, these tumors have atypical pleomorphic stromal cells and irregularly sized adipocytes involving the dermis; the proportion of mature adipocytic component can vary considerably. As a result, other mesenchymal tumors with pleomorphic stromal cells including pleomorphic fibromas, pleomorphic liposarcomas, and pleomorphic lipomas can be confused for this entity [47, 49, 50]. In addition, large lipomas can superficially involve the skin raising concern of a "lipoma-like" well-differentiated liposarcoma. Finally, dedifferentiated liposarcoma can involve the overlying skin on exceptional occasions and can be problematic to diagnosis if the fatty component is not sampled (i.e., small biopsy) and/or clinical history not provided.

As previously mentioned, virtually all atypical lipomatous tumors/well-differentiated liposarcoma/dedifferentiated liposarcoma have amplification of 12q13~15 region [13, 47, 51]. FISH is a proven technique to identify amplification in this region and can distinguish de differentiated and well-differentiated/atypical lipomatous tumors from other lipomatous tumors and fibrous tumors with pleomorphic cells. Immunohistochemistry for MDM2 and CDK4 (proteins from genes amplified in the 12q13~15 interval) have also been used to demonstrate overexpression. Different labs report variable levels of success with this approach.

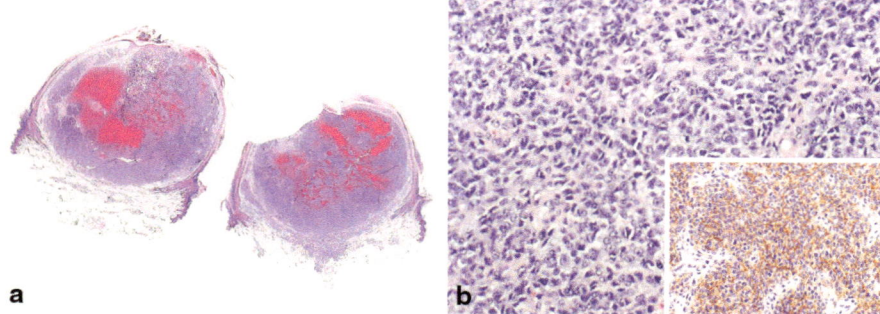

Fig. 3.6 Cutaneous Ewing sarcoma positive for *EWSR1-FLI1* fusion transcript by RT-PCR. **a** Low power. **b** High power with CD99 (inset).

Unusual Cutaneous Presentations of Mesenchymal Tumors

Mesenchymal tumor, which normally occurs in deep soft tissue or even the bone, can unexpectedly present superficially as a primary, metastases or extend to the skin [2]. A few examples of this include clear cell sarcoma (as previously discussed earlier), nodular fasciitis, rhabdomyosarcoma, synovial sarcoma, and Ewing sarcoma (see Figs. 3.6 & 3.7) [3, 52–54]. Although Ewing sarcoma is more commonly thought as a primary bone tumor, they can rarely occur as a primary cutaneous tumor and cause diagnostic confusion with melanoma, merkel cell carcinoma or even lymphoma. Like their deeper counterparts, these tumors are composed of small round cells which label for CD99 often with distinct membranous accentuation. Fortunately, these tumors have rearrangements involving *EWSR1* that can be detected by FISH or by RT-PCR assays. Synovial sarcoma can also occasionally be primary to the skin or involve the overlying dermis. The differential can include nerve sheath tumors and fibrosarcomatous transformation in DFSP. Synovial sarcoma will be positive for rearrangements involving *SS18* also known as *SYT* (18q11) [1]. RT-PCR assay is also available in most commercial testing laboratories, with most detecting *SYT-SSX1* and *SYT-SSX2*, the most common fusion transcript variants for synovial sarcoma, though *SSX4* can also rarely be involved.

Summary

Mesenchymal tumors presenting in the skin are uncommon to rare and can present unique challenges. However, a variety of molecular diagnostic tests are commercially available that can offer diagnostic assistance. Each of these tests has strengths and limitations that are important to consider when choosing which method is appropriate and how best to interpret the results to arrive at a diagnosis. New discoveries continue to expand our understanding of this tumor family, some of which can

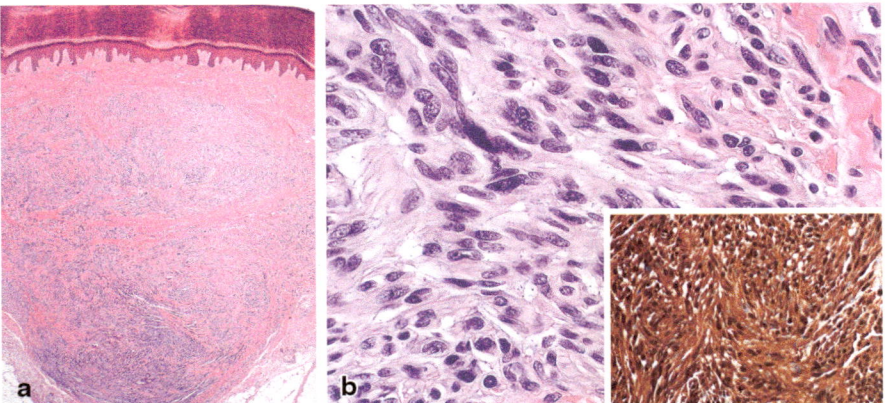

Fig. 3.7 Cutaneous clear cell sarcoma with *EWSR1* rearrangement. **a** Low power. **b** High power with S100 protein (inset).

be adapted to aid in diagnosis and possibly in the treatment of these tumors. As with the application of any molecular test, such information in dermal mesenchymal tumors must always be interpreted within the context of the clinical setting combined with morphologic and immunohistochemical features of the tumor. An informed, holistic view is the best approach for diagnosis with referral to expert consultants in highly unusual cases or in areas with diagnosis experience is extremely limited.

References

1. Fletcher CDM. World health organization. International agency for research on cancer. WHO classification of tumours of soft tissue and bone. 4th ed. Lyon: IARC Press; 2013.
2. Wang WL, Bones-Valentin RA, Prieto VG, Pollock RE, Lev DC, Lazar AJ. Sarcoma metastases to the skin: a clinicopathologic study of 65 patients. Cancer. 2012;118:2900–4.
3. Shingde MV, Buckland M, Busam KJ, McCarthy SW, Wilmott J, Thompson JF, et al. Primary cutaneous Ewing sarcoma/primitive neuroectodermal tumour: a clinicopathological analysis of seven cases highlighting diagnostic pitfalls and the role of FISH testing in diagnosis. J Clin Pathol. 2009;62:915–9.
4. Hantschke M, Mentzel T, Rutten A, Palmedo G, Calonje E, Lazar AJ, et al. Cutaneous clear cell sarcoma: a clinicopathologic, immunohistochemical, and molecular analysis of 12 cases emphasizing its distinction from dermal melanoma. Am J Surg Pathol. 2010;34:216–22.
5. Demicco EG, Lazar AJ. Clinicopathologic considerations: how can we fine tune our approach to sarcoma? Semin Oncol. 2011;38(Suppl 3):S3–S18.
6. Lazar AJ, Trent JC, Lev D. Sarcoma molecular testing: diagnosis and prognosis. Curr Oncol Rep. 2007;9:309–15.
7. Lessnick SL, Dei Tos AP, Sorensen PH, Dileo P, Baker LH, Ferrari S, et al. Small round cell sarcomas. Semin Oncol. 2009;36:338–46.
8. Hollmann TJ, Hornick JL. INI1-deficient tumors: diagnostic features and molecular genetics. Am J Surg Pathol. 2011;35:e47–e63.
9. Hornick JL, Dal Cin P, Fletcher CD. Loss of INI1 expression is characteristic of both conventional and proximal-type epithelioid sarcoma. Am J Surg Pathol. 2009;33:542–50.

10. Demetri GD, von Mehren M, Antonescu CR, DeMatteo RP, Ganjoo KN, Maki RG, et al. NCCN Task Force report: update on the management of patients with gastrointestinal stromal tumors. J Natl Compr Canc Netw. 2010;8(Suppl 2):S1–41; quiz S2–4.

11. Yang J, Du X, Lazar AJ, Pollock R, Hunt K, Chen K, et al. Genetic aberrations of gastrointestinal stromal tumors. Cancer. 2008;113:1532–43.

12. Lazar AJ, Tuvin D, Hajibashi S, Habeeb S, Bolshakov S, Mayordomo-Aranda E, et al. Specific mutations in the beta-catenin gene (CTNNB1) correlate with local recurrence in sporadic desmoid tumors. Am J Pathol. 2008;173:1518–27.

13. Weaver J, Downs-Kelly E, Goldblum JR, Turner S, Kulkarni S, Tubbs RR, et al. Fluorescence in situ hybridization for MDM2 gene amplification as a diagnostic tool in lipomatous neoplasms. Mod Pathol. 2008;21:943–9.

14. Boland JM, Folpe AL. Cutaneous neoplasms showing EWSR1 rearrangement. Adv Anat Pathol. 2013;20:75–85.

15. Fisher C. The diversity of soft tissue tumours with EWSR1 gene rearrangements: a review. Histopathology. 2014;64:134–50.

16. Rossi S, Szuhai K, Ijszenga M, Tanke HJ, Zanatta L, Sciot R, et al. EWSR1-CREB1 and EWSR1-ATF1 fusion genes in angiomatoid fibrous histiocytoma. Clin Cancer Res. 2007;13:7322–8.

17. Thway K, Fisher C. Tumors with EWSR1-CREB1 and EWSR1-ATF1 fusions: the current status. Am J Surg Pathol. 2012;36:e1–e11.

18. Wang WL, Mayordomo E, Zhang W, Hernandez VS, Tuvin D, Garcia L, et al. Detection and characterization of EWSR1/ATF1 and EWSR1/CREB1 chimeric transcripts in clear cell sarcoma (melanoma of soft parts). Mod Pathol. 2009;22:1201–9.

19. Antonescu CR, Dal Cin P, Nafa K, Teot LA, Surti U, Fletcher CD, et al. EWSR1-CREB1 is the predominant gene fusion in angiomatoid fibrous histiocytoma. Genes Chromosomes Cancer. 2007;46:1051–60.

20. Antonescu CR, Nafa K, Segal NH, Dal Cin P, Ladanyi M. EWS-CREB1: a recurrent variant fusion in clear cell sarcoma–association with gastrointestinal location and absence of melanocytic differentiation. Clin Cancer Res. 2006;12:5356–62.

21. Antonescu CR, Katabi N, Zhang L, Sung YS, Seethala RR, Jordan RC, et al. EWSR1-ATF1 fusion is a novel and consistent finding in hyalinizing clear-cell carcinoma of salivary gland. Genes Chromosom Cancer. 2011;50:559–70.

22. Yancoskie AE, Sreekantaiah C, Jacob J, Rosenberg A, Edelman M, Antonescu CR, et al. EWSR1 and ATF1 rearrangements in clear cell odontogenic carcinoma: presentation of a case. Oral Surg Oral Med Oral Pathol Oral Radiol. 2014;118:e115–8.

23. Thway K, Nicholson AG, Lawson K, Gonzalez D, Rice A, Balzer B, et al. Primary pulmonary myxoid sarcoma with EWSR1-CREB1 fusion: a new tumor entity. Am J Surg Pathol. 2011;35:1722–32.

24. Bilodeau EA, Weinreb I, Antonescu CR, Zhang L, Dacic S, Muller S, et al. Clear cell odontogenic carcinomas show EWSR1 rearrangements: a novel finding and a biological link to salivary clear cell carcinomas. Am J Surg Pathol. 2013;37:1001–5.

25. Mejia-Guerrero S, Quejada M, Gokgoz N, Gill M, Parkes RK, Wunder JS, et al. Characterization of the 12q15 MDM2 and 12q13-14 CDK4 amplicons and clinical correlations in osteosarcoma. Genes Chromosom Cancer. 2010;49:518–25.

26. Patel KU, Szabo SS, Hernandez VS, Prieto VG, Abruzzo LV, Lazar AJ, et al. Dermatofibrosarcoma protuberans COL1A1-PDGFB fusion is identified in virtually all dermatofibrosarcoma protuberans cases when investigated by newly developed multiplex reverse transcription polymerase chain reaction and fluorescence in situ hybridization assays. Hum Pathol. 2008;39:184–93.

27. Antonescu CR, Tschernyavsky SJ, Woodruff JM, Jungbluth AA, Brennan MF, Ladanyi M. Molecular diagnosis of clear cell sarcoma: detection of EWS-ATF1 and MITF-M transcripts and histopathological and ultrastructural analysis of 12 cases. J Mol Diagn. 2002;4:44–52.

28. Mentzel T, Scharer L, Kazakov DV, Michal M. Myxoid dermatofibrosarcoma protuberans: clinicopathologic, immunohistochemical, and molecular analysis of eight cases. Am J Dermatopathol. 2007;29:443–8.
29. Zelger BW, Ofner D, Zelger BG. Atrophic variants of dermatofibroma and dermatofibrosarcoma protuberans. Histopathology. 1995;26:519–27.
30. Mentzel T, Beham A, Katenkamp D, Dei Tos AP, Fletcher CD. Fibrosarcomatous ("high-grade") dermatofibrosarcoma protuberans: clinicopathologic and immunohistochemical study of a series of 41 cases with emphasis on prognostic significance. Am J Surg Pathol. 1998;22:576–87.
31. Swaby MG, Evans HL, Fletcher CD, Prieto VG, Patel KU, Lev DC, et al. Dermatofibrosarcoma protuberans with unusual sarcomatous transformation: a series of 4 cases with molecular confirmation. Am J Dermatopathol. 2011;33:354–60.
32. Wang WL, Patel KU, Coleman NM, Smith-Zagone MJ, Ivan D, Reed JA, et al. COL1A1:PDGFB chimeric transcripts are not present in indeterminate fibrohistiocytic lesions of the skin. Am J Dermatopathol. 2010;32:149–53.
33. Kutzner H, Mentzel T, Palmedo G, Hantschke M, Rutten A, Paredes BE, et al. Plaque-like CD34-positive dermal fibroma ("medallion-like dermal dendrocyte hamartoma"): clinicopathologic, immunohistochemical, and molecular analysis of 5 cases emphasizing its distinction from superficial, plaque-like dermatofibrosarcoma protuberans. Am J Surg Pathol. 2010;34:190–201.
34. Weaver J, Billings SD. Postradiation cutaneous vascular tumors of the breast: a review. Semin Diagn Pathol. 2009;26:141–9.
35. Flucke U, Requena L, Mentzel T. Radiation-induced vascular lesions of the skin: an overview. Adv Anat Pathol. 2013;20:407–15.
36. Fernandez AP, Sun Y, Tubbs RR, Goldblum JR, Billings SD. FISH for MYC amplification and anti-MYC immunohistochemistry: useful diagnostic tools in the assessment of secondary angiosarcoma and atypical vascular proliferations. J Cutan Pathol. 2012;39:234–42.
37. Mentzel T, Schildhaus HU, Palmedo G, Buttner R, Kutzner H. Postradiation cutaneous angiosarcoma after treatment of breast carcinoma is characterized by MYC amplification in contrast to atypical vascular lesions after radiotherapy and control cases: clinicopathological, immunohistochemical and molecular analysis of 66 cases. Mod Pathol. 2012;25:75–85.
38. Billings SD, Folpe AL, Weiss SW. Epithelioid Sarcoma-like hemangioendothelioma (pseudomyogenic hemangioendothelioma). Am J Surg Pathol. 2011;35:1088; author reply—9.
39. Hornick JL, Fletcher CD. Pseudomyogenic hemangioendothelioma: a distinctive, often multicentric tumor with indolent behavior. Am J Surg Pathol. 2011;35:190–201.
40. Walther C, Tayebwa J, Lilljebjorn H, Magnusson L, Nilsson J, von Steyern FV, et al. A novel SERPINE1-FOSB fusion gene results in transcriptional up-regulation of FOSB in pseudomyogenic haemangioendothelioma. J Pathol. 2014;232:534–40.
41. Antonescu CR, Zhang L, Chang NE, Pawel BR, Travis W, Katabi N, et al. EWSR1-POU5F1 fusion in soft tissue myoepithelial tumors. A molecular analysis of sixty-six cases, including soft tissue, bone, and visceral lesions, showing common involvement of the EWSR1 gene. Genes Chromosom Cancer. 2010;49:1114–24.
42. Agaram NP, Chen HW, Zhang L, Sung YS, Panicek D, Healey JH, et al. EWSR1-PBX3: a novel gene fusion in myoepithelial tumors. Genes Chromosom Cancer. 2015;54:63–71.
43. Huang SC, Chen HW, Zhang L, Sung YS, Agaram NP, Davis M, et al. Novel FUS-KLF17 and EWSR1-KLF17 fusions in myoepithelial tumors. Genes Chromosom Cancer. 2015;54(5):267–75.
44. Antonescu CR, Zhang L, Shao SY, Mosquera JM, Weinreb I, Katabi N, et al. Frequent PLAG1 gene rearrangements in skin and soft tissue myoepithelioma with ductal differentiation. Genes Chromosom Cancer. 2013;52:675–82.
45. Wang WL, Mayordomo E, Czerniak BA, Abruzzo LV, Dal Cin P, Araujo DM, et al. Fluorescence in situ hybridization is a useful ancillary diagnostic tool for extraskeletal myxoid chondrosarcoma. Mod Pathol. 2008;21:1303–10.

46. Paredes BE, Mentzel T. Atypical lipomatous tumor/"well-differentiated liposarcoma" of the skin clinically presenting as a skin tag: clinicopathologic, immunohistochemical, and molecular analysis of 2 cases. Am J Dermatopathol. 2011;33:603–7.

47. Al-Zaid T, Wang WL, Lopez-Terrada D, Lev D, Hornick JL, Hafeez Diwan A, et al. Pleomorphic fibroma and dermal atypical lipomatous tumor: are they related? J Cutan Pathol. 2013;40:379–84.

48. Dei Tos AP, Mentzel T, Fletcher CD. Primary liposarcoma of the skin: a rare neoplasm with unusual high grade features. Am J Dermatopathol. 1998;20:332–8.

49. Sachdeva MP, Goldblum JR, Rubin BP, Billings SD. Low-fat and fat-free pleomorphic lipomas: a diagnostic challenge. Am J Dermatopathol. 2009;31:423–6.

50. Gardner JM, Dandekar M, Thomas D, Goldblum JR, Weiss SW, Billings SD, et al. Cutaneous and subcutaneous pleomorphic liposarcoma: a clinicopathologic study of 29 cases with evaluation of MDM2 gene amplification in 26. Am J Surg Pathol. 2012;36:1047–51.

51. Tanas MR, Rubin BP, Tubbs RR, Billings SD, Downs-Kelly E, Goldblum JR. Utilization of fluorescence in situ hybridization in the diagnosis of 230 mesenchymal neoplasms: an institutional experience. Arch Pathol Lab Med. 2010;134:1797–803.

52. Marburger TB, Gardner JM, Prieto VG, Billings SD. Primary cutaneous rhabdomyosarcoma: a clinicopathologic review of 11 cases. J Cutan Pathol. 2012;39:987–95.

53. Fletcher CD, McKee PH. Sarcomas–a clinicopathological guide with particular reference to cutaneous manifestation. III. Angiosarcoma, malignant haemangiopericytoma, fibrosarcoma and synovial sarcoma. Clin Exp Dermatol. 1985;10:332–49.

54. Ehrig T, Billings SD, Fanburg-Smith JC. Superficial primitive neuroectodermal tumor/Ewing sarcoma (PN/ES): same tumor as deep PN/ES or new entity? Ann Diagn Pathol. 2007;11:153–9.

Chapter 4
Molecular Pathology of Cutaneous Adnexal Tumors

Doina Ivan and Phyu P. Aung

Introduction

Most of the cutaneous adnexal neoplasms are solitary and appear de novo. However, several entities have been described being associated with inherited syndromes and visceral neoplasms, frequently involving multiple organs. Considering that in some cases the first manifestation of an inherited syndrome or internal malignancy may be a cutaneous adnexal neoplasm, their early and correct recognition is of outmost importance for patient's follow-up, prognosis, and therapeutic options. In certain instances, the presence of a cutaneous adnexal neoplasm is considered patognomonic for a syndrome and has well-characterized genetic alterations implicated in the syndrome's pathogenesis.

As a general rule, cutaneous adnexal neoplasms associated with hereditary conditions or syndromes are multiple and often share similar histopathologic features with their sporadic counterparts. However, some lesions may provide histologic clues that suggest an associated syndrome and these characteristics are discussed further. Majority of the cutaneous adnexal tumors in syndromic settings are benign but malignant tumors can also occur. Interestingly, benign cutaneous adnexal tumors are frequently associated with malignant internal neoplasms. Most of the syndromes do not have genotype–phenotype correlation in terms of extent of cutaneous involvement or possibility of a malignant transformation.

The autosomal dominant pattern of inheritance is the most common mode of transmission of these conditions and is frequently characterized by a single gene locus alteration, usually involving tumor suppressor genes. This chapter provides a detailed description of these genetic alterations. Cutaneous adnexal tumors that may be potentially associated with a hereditary condition will be further described and

D. Ivan (✉) · P. P. Aung
Section of Dermatopathology, Department of Pathology, The University of Texas MD Anderson Cancer Center, Houston, TX 77030, USA
e-mail: dsivan@mdanderson@org

© Springer Science+Business Media New York 2015
V. G. Prieto (ed.), *Precision Molecular Pathology of Dermatologic Diseases,*
Molecular Pathology Library 9, DOI 10.1007/978-1-4939-2861-3_4

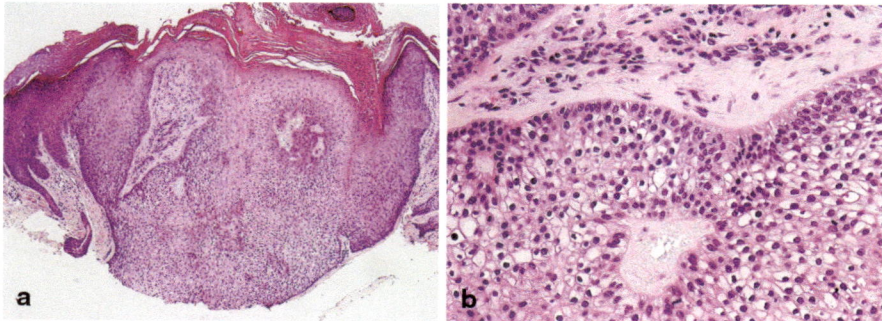

Fig. 4.1 Trichilemmoma—The histology shows lobular, folliculocentric proliferations of uniform, bland basaloid cells with peripheral palisading and frequent clear cell cytoplasm (due to PAS-positive glycogen accumulation) (**a**). A distinctive feature is the presence of a thick eosinophilic basal membrane (**b**)

categorized based on their type of adnexal differentiation: follicular, sweat gland, or sebaceous origin.

Molecular Alterations in Cutaneous Adnexal Tumors with Follicular Origin

Trichilemmoma

Clinical Features

Trichilemmoma is a relatively common cutaneous adnexal tumor derived from the follicular outer root sheath cells. It may be solitary or multiple and usually presents as a single, small, skin-colored papule on the face (nose and eyelids) of adult individuals [1].

Histology

Histologically, trichilemmomas are lobular, folliculocentric proliferations of uniform, bland basaloid cells with peripheral palisading and frequent clear cell cytoplasm (due to periodic acid–Schiff (PAS)-positive glycogen accumulation). A distinctive feature is the presence of a thick eosinophilic basal membrane (Fig. 4.1a, b). Overlying hyperkeratosis, parakeratosis, and focal squamous eddies formation may be noted [1, 2]. A distinctive variant is desmoplastic trichilemmoma that has a focally infiltrative growth pattern, associated desmoplastic stroma, and may mimic histologically invasive squamous cell carcinoma.

If solitary trichilemmomas are relatively common, multiple lesions are almost invariably associated with Cowden syndrome. Interestingly, the desmoplastic variant of trichilemmoma is not reported as being associated with Cowden syndrome [3].

Cowden Syndrome

Cowden syndrome (multiple hamartoma syndrome), originally described in 1963 by Lloyd and Dennis, is a multisystem hamartomatous disorder with associated macrocephaly, predominately affecting women [3]. The mucocutaneous manifestations of this syndrome are represented by multiple trichilemommas, predominately in the head and neck area, as well as by punctate acral keratoses of soles and hands, sclerotic fibromas, acrochordons, oral papillomas, and acrokeratosis verruciformis [4–8]. Mucocutaneous lesions are almost always identified in Cowden syndrome, are estimated to have 99 % penetrance by the 3rd decade of life, and may represent occasionally the first manifestation of Cowden syndrome [4].

Gastrointestinal polyps are present in 60–90 % of patients and benign thyroid lesions (adenomas, hamartomas, multinodular goiter, and Hashimoto thyroiditis) occur in up to 75 % of patients [9–11]. Benign breast lesions, genitourinary malformations, leiomyomas, lipomas, and vascular malformations are also described [11–13].

Most importantly, these patients have an increased risk for developing internal malignancies, mostly breast adenocarcinoma and thyroid carcinoma (usually follicular variant), gastrointestinal and genitourinary tumors, melanoma, etc [14, 15]. According to the literature reports, the lifetime risk for patients with Cowden syndrome is 85.2 % for breast carcinoma (as compared with 11 % within the general population), 35.2 % for thyroid carcinoma, 33.6 % for renal cell carcinoma, 28.2 % for endometrial carcinoma, 9 % for colonic carcinoma, and 6 % for melanoma [15]. As with other hereditary breast cancer syndromes, the breast adenocarcinoma in patients with Cowden syndrome occurs at a younger age (average 36–46 years) and male patients are also at risk of developing breast cancer [16].

Cowden syndrome is an autosomal dominant condition and is caused by a germline inactivating mutation in the tumor suppressor phosphatase and tensine homolog gene (PTEN) situated on chromosome 10q23.31 [17, 18]. PTEN is a tumor suppressor gene and is an important mediator of carcinogenesis in a variety of human malignancies [19–22]. PTEN is involved in apoptosis and cell cycle arrest and negatively regulates the cell survival and PI3K/Akt/mTOR pathway through its phosphatase activity. PTEN phosphatase uses Akt-activator phosphatidylinositol-3,4,5-triphosphate (PIP3) as a substrate [17, 21–23]. Moreover, PTEN negatively affects the mitogen-activated protein (MAP) pathway. It has been demonstrated that 80–85 % patients with Cowden syndrome have germline loss-of-function PTEN mutation, with approximately 40–60 % of cases estimated to be familial [24]. Frameshift, nonsense, and missense point mutations, deletions, insertions, and splice site mutations have been described. It was reported that although these mutations may be identified almost in the entire length of PTEN gene (with exception of first, fourth, and last exon), approximately half of the mutations were identified in exon 5, coding for the core phosphatase domain, which is responsible for phospholipid binding. Interestingly, a correlation was observed between the presence of PTEN mutation and breast adenocarcinoma [24]. Promoter mutations were associated with breast cancer, whereas colorectal carcinoma was associated with nonsense mutations.

Other mechanisms of PTEN loss-of-function, such as PTEN promoter hypermethylation (which leads to underexpression of PTEN) or PTEN inactivation through ubiquitin protein-mediated degradation, may account for the remainder cases [25]. Recently, PI3KCA and Akt1 germline mutations were reported in some patients with Cowden syndrome lacking PTEN mutations [26]. Also, germline epigenetic regulation of KILLIN was described in a subset of patients with Cowden or Cowden-like syndrome lacking germline PTEN mutations [27, 28]. KILLIN is identified as a TP53 regulated inhibitor of DNA synthesis through S phase arrest, is transcribed in the opposite (i.e., antisense) strand relative to PTEN, and shares the same promoter region as PTEN. It has been reported that individuals with KILLIN-promoter hypermethylation have a threefold increased prevalence in breast cancer and a greater than twofold increase in kidney cancer prevalence over individuals with germline PTEN mutations [28].

As a practical approach for a patient in which more than one trichilemmoma was histologically diagnosed, a difference in expression of PREN by immunohistochemistry in patients with Cowden syndrome versus sporadic cases was shown recently. It is reported that complete PTEN loss in trichilemmomas by immunohistochemistry is strongly suggestive of association with Cowden syndrome, but retention of PTEN labeling does not entirely exclude the syndrome [29].

A heterogenous group of individuals with Cowden-like syndrome, but not meeting Cowden syndrome inclusion criteria such as presence of PTEN germline mutation, is increasingly recognized. There are pathognomonic diagnostic criteria for the diagnosis of Cowden syndrome, updated annually by the US National Comprehensive Cancer Network.

PTEN hamartoma tumor syndrome (PHTS) is a term encompassing subsets of several clinical syndromes with germline mutations in PTEN tumor suppressor gene. These syndromes have autosomal dominant transmission with variable phenotypic manifestations and are characterized by germline mutations of PTEN located at 10q22–23 [17, 21–23]. Cowden syndrome is the prototypic PHTS but this category also includes: Lhermitte–Duclos disease, Bannayan–Riley–Ruvalcaba syndrome, and possibly Proteus syndrome. Lhermitte–Duclos disease is characterized by dysplastic gangliocytoma of the cerebellum which leads to increase in intracranial pressure, ataxia, and seizures. Bannayan–Riley–Ruvalcaba syndrome presents with developmental delay, macrocephaly, lipomas, hemangiomas, and pigmented penile speckled macules. Proteus syndrome is a rapidly progressive disorder characterized by mosaicism, congenital malformations, tissue overgrowth, epidermal nevi, hyperostosis, and various vascular anomalies. Notably, an increased risk for malignancy was demonstrated only for Cowden syndrome in the PHTS group [17, 22].

Clinical Management

Considering the increased risk of developing malignancies in Cowden Syndrome, the most critical aspect is close and heightened cancer surveillance. As a general rule, any patient who meets the patognomonic criteria for Cowden syndrome is indicated to be referred to genetic counseling, and sequencing of PTEN should be considered [9]. There is no definite consensus regarding the patients with Cowden-like syndrome, but not meeting the inclusion criteria [4]. Screening for breast cancer is indicated to start at an earlier age (30–35 years) and includes annual mammograms and magnetic resonance imaging (MRI), but there is also an increased concern that this will lead to a high degree of false-positive data and a high yield of unnecessary procedures. Total thyroidectomy is generally recommended in patients who develop thyroid cancer because of a high risk of recurrence. The current guidelines also recommend annual endometrial biopsies for premenopausal women and endometrial ultrasound for postmenopausal women [4, 17, 22].

The development of PI3K/Akt/mTOR inhibitors is extensively studied in oncology, as this pathway promotes cellular survival and chemotherapeutic resistance in a variety of malignancies. mTOR inhibitors are especially promising in patients with Cowden syndrome [17].

Pilomatricoma ("Calcifying Epithelioma of Malherbe")

Clinical Features

Pilomatricoma is a relatively common skin adnexal tumor with follicular origin and differentiation toward the follicular matrix, which mimics in its evolution the hair growth. It predominately affects children and young adults, more than half of the cases developing in the first 2 decades of life, and has a 3:1 female preponderance. It usually involves the head, neck, and upper extremities, and less frequently trunk and lower extremities [30–33]. Pilomatricoma presents as frequently solitary well-circumscribed, firm, slow-growing, asymptomatic, 1–3 cm in maximum dimension, deep dermal or subcutaneous nodules covered with normal skin tissue. Rarely, variants of pilomatricomas were described: perforating, exophytic, multinodular, giant, and bullous clinical types [30–33].

Histology

The histologic features of pilomatricoma depend on its stage of development. Early lesions are frequently cystic with areas resembling a follicular cyst, infundibular type, areas containing basaloid cells resembling the follicular metrical cells (hyperchromatic nuclei, high nuclear/cytoplasmic ratio, and numerous mitotic figures) and supramatrical cells with eosinophilic cytoplasm, without nuclear structures (called

Fig. 4.2 Pilomatricoma—
The histologic features reveal
areas containing basaloid
cells resembling the follicular
matrical cells (hyperchromatic nuclei, high nuclear/
cytoplasmic ratio, and
numerous mitotic figures)
and supramatrical cells with
eosinophilic cytoplasm,
without nuclear structures
(shadow or ghosts cells)

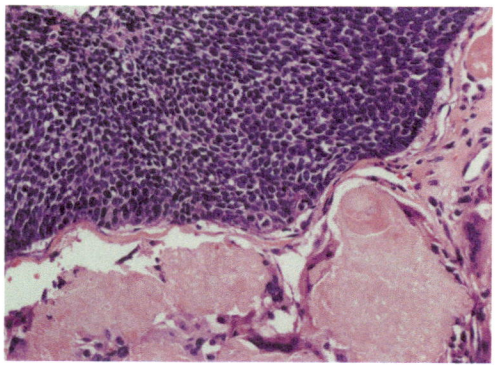

shadow or ghosts cells). (Fig. 4.2) As the lesion progresses, the shadow cells predominate whereas the metrical cells become less obvious. Dystrophic calcifications
and metaplastic ossification are commonly seen in this stage. Late-stage lesions can
occasionally imitate osteomas.

If solitary pilomatricoma is very common, multiple pilomatricomas (usually up
to 5) can be found in conjunction with a variety of abnormalities including myotonic dystrophy, Turner's syndrome, trisomy 9, Gardner's syndrome, Sotos syndrome,
Rubinsten–Taybi syndrome, etc. [34–37].

Current studies have revealed that sporadic pilomatricomas have activation mutations in the cytoskeletal and cell-signaling protein β-catenin, encoded by *CTNNB1*
gene located on the 3p22–p21.3 region [38–42]. β-catenin is a 92-kDa protein involved in both WNT-signaling pathway and intercellular adhesion. It is suggested
that WNT/β-catenin/LEF (lymphoid enhancer factor) pathway is activated in normal hair follicular matrix to induce differentiation toward hair shaft [43]. Activated
WNT signaling leads to suppression of β-catenin phosphorylation and accumulated
protein translocates to the nucleus, where it acts along with LEF to activate various transcription genes, such as *MYC*, *CYC D1*, etc. [44]. Nuclear accumulation of
β-catenin can be demonstrated by using immunohistochemical studies and suggests
either an activation of WNT-signaling pathway or a mutation that reduces β-catenin
phosphorylation. Presence of β-catenin in the nucleus promotes cellular proliferation and was demonstrated in other tumors, such as colorectal carcinomas, melanoma, endometrial, pancreatic, and hepatocellular carcinomas [40, 45]. Mutations in
CTNNB1 are located in the exon 3 region of the gene, which encodes the N-terminal
phosphorylation sites. Missense mutations at these sites lead to β-catenin stabiliza-
tion through decreased phosphorylation and degradation. In the skin, apart from
pilomatricomas, mutations in exon 3 of CTNNB1 gene were also found in other
tumors such as trichoepithelioma, basal cell carcinoma, and pilomatrical carcinoma,
suggesting that β-catenin gene mutations contribute to these tumors tumorigenesis
[40, 42, 45]. By immunohistochemistry, nuclear β-catenin, nuclear Lef-1, and cyclin
D1 can be detected in the basaloid cells of pilomatricoma and pilomatrix carcinoma.

The role of bcl-2 in the histogenesis of pilomatricoma was recently reported
[46]. *Bcl-2* gene, located on chromosome 18, encodes an oncoprotein that blocks

the apoptosis not only in various cells, such as lymphocytes, but also in the matrical follicular cells.

Fibrofolliculoma/Trichodiscoma

Clinical Features

Fibrofolliculoma and fibrodiscoma are follicular-derived benign cutaneous tumors, currently considered by many as part of the same histologic spectrum. They present as asymptomatic, small (1–4 mm), white-skin colored smooth papules. They are commonly found on the neck, upper chest, upper back, and face [47]. The lesions may range from one to several hundreds over a lifetime [48]. Fibrofolliculomas normally appear in the third and fourth decade of life (median age of 54 years) with no predilection for either sex [48]. The number and size of the fibrofolliculomas may increase with age; in cases with multiple lesions, they have the potential to be disfiguring, causing psychological burden [49].

Histopathology

Histopathologically, as the name suggests, fibrofolliculoma is a benign hamartomatous lesion with combined features of proliferation of hair follicle and perifollicular fibrous tissue. There are strands and cords of epithelial cells that are 2–4 cells thick, radiating from the infundibulum of a follicle that may be dilated and filled with keratinous material. The strands are surrounded by loose connective tissue containing fine collagen fibers with intervening mucin and partial or complete loss of elastic fibers. The epithelial strands may anastomose with each other or unite with the follicular infundibulum [50] (Fig. 4.3).

On the other hand, trichodiscoma is a well circumscribed but nonencapsulated benign tumor with overlying flattened epidermis and folliculosebaceous units

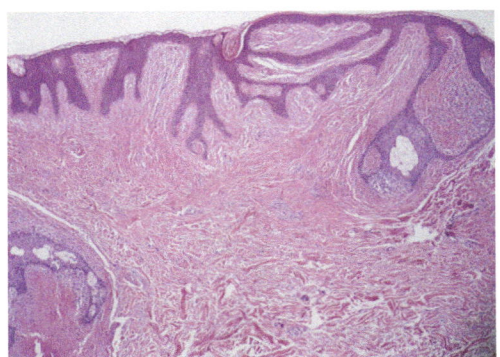

Fig. 4.3 Fibrofolliculoma— Histologically characterized by anastomosing strands and cords of epithelial cells radiating from the follicular infundibulum and surrounded by loose connective tissue with partial or complete loss of elastic fibers

forming a collarette. It is composed of loosely arranged fascicles of fine collagen fibers intermingled with spindle-to-stellate-shaped fibroblasts in a background of mucinous stroma. There may be admixed prominent small blood vessels with PAS-positive basement membranes and few nerve fibers, predominantly at the periphery of the lesion [50].

Birt–Hogg–Dubé Syndrome (BHDS)

BHDS is a rare autosomal dominant inherited genodermatosis [48, 51]. BHDS is named after three authors (Canadian physicians Birt, Hogg, and Dube) who published a paper in 1977 describing family members with papular skin lesions on their face, forehead, scalp, and neck [50]. These three skin lesions characteristic of BHDS are fibrofolliculoma, trichodiscoma, and acrochordon. Acrochordon are very common lesions in general population and are rarely associated with BHDS [52, 53]. In one study, cutaneous lesions were found in 90 % (46/51) of families with BHDS [47]. For unknown reasons, Asian patients with BHDS are less likely to develop the cutaneous manifestations of the disease [54].

In addition to this skin lesion, people with BHDS are at increased risk of developing lung cysts, spontaneous pneumothorax, and kidney neoplasms [48]. Patients with fibrofolliculomas have a 50-fold increased risk for developing spontaneous pneumothorax, and a 7-fold increased risk for renal carcinoma [55]. It is important to recognize the possible association between fibrofolliculomas and BHDS as the diagnosis of the cutaneous lesion may lead to the early detection of life-threatening conditions, such as kidney neoplasms and pneumothorax. In one study, 72 % (18/25) families with kidney tumors were diagnosed after recruiting based on cutaneous manifestations of fibrofolliculoma [47].

Molecular Findings

In 2001, a BHD-associated gene locus was localized to chromosome 17p11.2 by linkage analysis [56]. Subsequently, truncating germline mutations were identified in a novel gene, the *FLCN* (BHD) gene (GenBank accession number AF517523), coding for a protein of unknown function [57]. The *FLCN* gene contains 14 exons and encodes folliculin, an evolutionary conserved protein of 579 aminoacids, with a central glutamic acid-rich coiled-coil domain, one N-glycosylation site, and three myristoylation sites, which has no major homology to any other human protein [58]. The function of folliculin is largely unknown. Somatic second-hit mutations in *FLCN*, identified in BHD-associated renal tumors, are consistent with a tumor suppressor function [59]. Loss of *FLCN* mRNA expression was found in renal tumors from patients with BHD, however, *FLCN* mRNA was reported to be strongly expressed in fibrofolliculomas. Loss of heterozygosity was not detected in fibrofolliculomas, suggesting that haploinsufficiency is sufficient to cause benign tumor growth in the skin and the mechanisms of tumorigenesis might differ in renal and skin tumors [60].

The mTOR (mammalian/mechanistic target of rapamycin complex 1) pathway, a key regulator of cell growth, proliferation, and metabolism, has been proposed to be involved in the pathogenesis of several hereditary hamartoma syndromes, including BHD. The precise role of *FLCN* in the mTOR pathway requires further elucidation, since several publications have reported contradictory effects of *FLCN* and it seems likely that *FLCN* has several functions. There are reports proposing that mTOR pathway is regulated by the interaction of *FLCN* and AMPK (5′AMP-activated protein kinase) mediated by FNIP1, a 130-kDa *FLCN*-interacting protein and FNIP2, an FNIP homologue [61, 62]. However, in a clinical trial, topical use of the mTOR inhibitor rapamycin was not an effective treatment for fibrofolliculo-mas [49]. *FLCN* may also be involved in the regulation of the TGF-beta signaling pathway, by deactivation of the transcription factor TFE3, and in overexpression of nuclear genes involved in the transcription and replication of the mitochondrial genome [63]. It has also been suggested that Drosophila BHD homolog (DBHD) may regulate maintenance of germline stem cells, downstream of, or in parallel with the JAK/STAT (which is necessary for germline stem cell self-renewal) and Dpp (a TGF-beta family member) signaling pathways [64]. Clarifying the roles of *FLCN* in the molecular pathogenesis of BHD-associated diseases might lead to the development of targeted therapies.

A germline *FLCN* mutation was found, by sequence analysis, in 84–88% of families with BHD and 3–5% of families had partial- or whole-gene deletions identified by other methods [47, 51]. Most of the reported pathogenic *FLCN* mutations are frameshift (52.9%, 37/70) or nonsense mutations (10/70, 14.3%) that lead to protein truncation, and followed by splice-site alterations (14/70, 20%) [65]. The majority of mutations are deletions (45%), substitutions (32–36%), duplications (15%), insertion/deletions (6%), and insertions (2%) [65, 66]. To date, the *FCLN* database includes more than 80 variants with > 53 unique germline mutations and > 30 SNPs. The unique germline BHD mutations have been reported in translated exons (4–14, excluding 8 and 10) of the BHD gene [47, 51]. The most frequent mutation in BHD patients is the insertion or deletion of a cytosine in the mononucleotide tract of eight cytosines (C8) in exon 11, predicted to cause a frameshift and prematurely truncate the mutant protein. This hot spot mutation occurs in about half of all BHD patients. Very few missense *FLCN* mutations were reported (e.g., 1523A→G [Lys508Arg]) [47, 51]. Mutations are located along the entire length of the coding region, with no genotype–phenotype correlations noted between type of mutation, location within the gene, and phenotypic disease manifestations [47].

The identification of *FLCN* defects in families with BHDS has led to a more accurate diagnosis. Formerly, BHDS was defined by the presence of multiple fibrofolliculomas (at least 5–10); the current proposed diagnostic criteria are based on clinical manifestations and the outcome of DNA testing [48, 56]. Patients should fulfill one major or two minor criteria of the following: Two major criteria are: (1) at least five fibrofolliculomas/trichodiscomas, at least one histologically confirmed, of adult onset and (2) pathogenic *FLCN* germline mutation. The three minor criteria are: (1) multiple lung cysts: bilateral basally located lung cysts with no other apparent cause, with or without spontaneous primary pneumothorax, (2) renal cancer, early onset

(<50 years) or multifocal or bilateral renal cancer, or renal cancer of mixed chromophobe and oncocytic histology, and (3) a first-degree relative with BHD [67].

Genetic Testing

FLCN is currently the only gene known to be associated with BHD. An MLPA (multiplex ligation-dependent probe amplification) kit for *FLCN* deletion and amplification analysis is available for genetic testing. The *FLCN* mutation database has been established by Wei and colleagues (http://www.skingenedatabase.com) and by the European BHD Consortium (Folliculin Sequence Variation Database). Mutation detection should be recommended for confirmation of diagnosis in suspected patients, as well as presymptomatic testing of at-risk relatives. Given the variable clinical manifestations of BHDS, genetic testing plays an important role in the identification of affected family members without skin tumors that could be at risk for developing renal tumors. The offspring of an individual with BHDS has a 50 % chance of inheriting the pathogenic variant (autosomal dominant) and prenatal diagnosis is possible if the *FLCN* pathogenic variant of an affected family member has been identified.

As per NCI recommendation, genetic testing for molecular diagnosis of a proband suspected of having BHDS should begin by sequence analysis of exon 11, as majority of the affected individuals have one of the two pathogenic variants found in exon 11. If a pathologic variant is not identified in exon 11, sequencing of the entire coding region of *FLCN* should be considered. If full-gene sequence analysis does not identify a pathogenic variant, deletion/duplication analysis of *FLCN* may be considered. Multigene panel by whole-exome sequencing may be considered in individuals with a clinical diagnosis of BHDS, but in whom no pathogenic variant in *FLCN* is identified. Surveillance in *FLCN*-mutation carriers and presymptomatic testing of family members of a confirmed BHD patient usually begins at the age of 18–20 years to allow counseling and informed consent before genetic testing, respectively. However, earlier testing and surveillance might be indicated in the families with a history of very early onset of pneumothorax or renal cancer [67].

Molecular Alterations in Cutaneous Adnexal Tumors with Sweat Gland Origin

Cylindroma/Spiradenoma

Clinical Features

Cylindromas and spiradenomas are difficult to distinguish clinically; they occur predominately in the head and neck region and present as multiple skin-colored small papules [68]. Spiradenoma can have a distinctive blue color and can also be painful [69]. The tumors appear early in adulthood and gradually increase in size and number throughout life, and may cause considerable disfigurement and discomfort.

Brooke–Spiegler syndrome (BSS) is an autosomal dominant disorder that predisposes affected patients to benign adnexal neoplasms including cylindromas, trichoepitheliomas, and/or spiradenomas. Ancell–Spiegler cylindromas (inherited disease of cylindromas) and Brooke–Fordyce trichoepitheliomas (inherited disease of trichoepitheliomas) were separate disorders first recognized in the mid-1800s [70–73]. With subsequent reports of the occurrence of trichoepitheliomas and cylindromas in the same patients, it became clear that these tumors were genetically related and the term BSS is now used for patients with multiple cylindromas, trichoeptheliomas, or a combination of both [69]. Some of the patients also develop spiradenomas, hence the triad of skin neoplasms (cylindromas, trichoepitheliomas, and/or spiradenomas) became characteristic of BSS [74].

Any or all of these tumors may develop at any point in life and there is variable penetrance within affected families [75]. Malignant transformation of these tumors is rare, but some studies suggest that tumors occurring in the setting of BSS can be more aggressive than their sporadic counterparts [76, 77]. Although BSS is inherited in autosomal dominant pattern, there is reduced penetrance in males with cylindromas and trichoepitheliomas occurring more commonly in females [78].

Histological Features

Cylindromas and spiradenomas are considered as being part of the same histologic spectrum and are tumors with eccrine or apocrine differentiation [79]. Trichoepitheliomas are follicular-derived lesions.

Cylindromas are histologically characterized by a dermal nodule composed of irregularly arranged islands of basaloid cells, sometimes admixed with small duct-like structures, surrounded by a thin eosinophilic band of hyaline material, arranged in a characteristic "jigsaw puzzle" pattern [80]. Most of the tumor islands show two cell types: a peripheral cell with a palisading dark-staining nucleus and a more centrally located larger cell with a vesicular nucleus. Both cell types are embedded in a stroma with loose collagen containing an increased number of fibroblasts. (Fig. 4.4)

Trichoepitheliomas are dermal tumors showing focal continuity with the epidermis in up to one third of cases. They are composed of uniform basaloid cells with peripheral palisades, arranged in variably sized nests or with a cribriform pattern, surrounded by dense stroma and fibroblasts [81]. Epithelial structures resembling hair papillae or abortive hair follicles (papillary mesenchymal bodies) and small keratinous cysts lined by stratified squamous epithelium may be seen. The desmoplastic trichoepithelioma variant is histologically characterized by a dense and hypocellular stroma, with fewer elastic fibers and more acid mucopolysaccharides.

Spiradenomas are dermal tumor nodules formed by nests of two types of epithelial cells arranged in cords, with tubular or alveolar differentiation, embedded in a background of edematous and vascular stroma [82]. The two cell types comprise

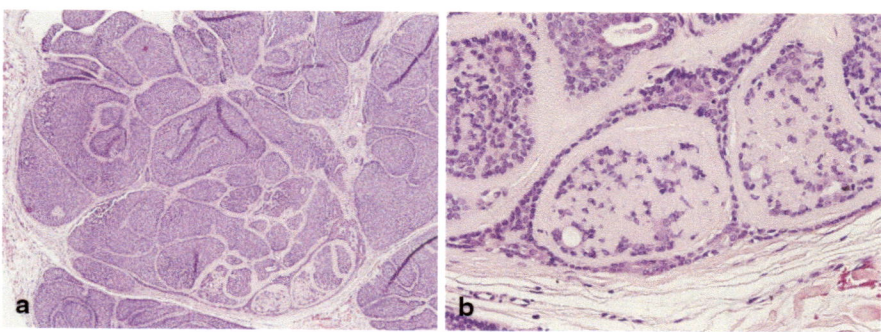

Fig. 4.4 Cylindroma/spiradenoma—Histologically characterized by a dermal nodule composed of "jigsaw puzzle"—arranged islands of basaloid cells with small duct-like structures, surrounded by an eosinophilic hyaline material (**a**). There are two cell types: a peripheral cell with a palisading dark-staining nucleus, and a more centrally located larger cell with a vesicular nucleus (**b**)

small dark basaloid cells with hyperchromatic nuclei and a more frequent larger cell with a pale nucleus (usually located in the center of the clusters). The cells are PAS negative, but droplets of PAS-positive hyaline material may be present in some areas. Duct-like structures, infiltrating lymphocytes, and irregular, thin fibrous bands containing blood vessels are often present within the tumor lobules.

Brooke–Spiegler Syndrome

Linkage analysis in families with multiple cylindromas first mapped the susceptibility gene to a single locus on chromosome 16q12–q13 [83, 84]. The *CYLD* gene was identified by positional cloning and germline mutations subsequently found in affected families [85]. The *CYLD* gene consists of 20 exons, of which the first three are untranslated (GenBank NM-015247). It encodes a 956 amino acid protein with a molecular weight of approximately 120 kDa. The mutations are scattered throughout the midportion and C-terminal region of the *CYLD* gene with 60 % clustering in the C-terminal region (exons 16–20), but not limited to one particular domain. The *CYLD* gene encodes the cylindromatosis protein (CYLD) (GenBank NP_056062), also known as ubiquitin-specific-processing protease CYLD, and ubiquitin carboxyl-terminal hydrolase CYLD. CYLD has moderate homology with proteins of the ubiquitin-specific protease class and it has enzymatic deubiquitinase activity. CYLD regulates cell functions including inflammation and cell proliferation through removal of ubiquitin of target proteins [86].

A total of 51 distinct germline *CYLD* mutations have been reported in the literature. The majority of the mutations are frameshift (41 %, 21/51) and nonsense (35 %, 18/51), followed by missense (14 %, 7/51), and putative splice site (10 %, 5/51) [86]. Eighty-six percent (44/51) of the mutations are predicted to result in truncated proteins. The most common reported mutation in *CYLD* is c.2806C > T,

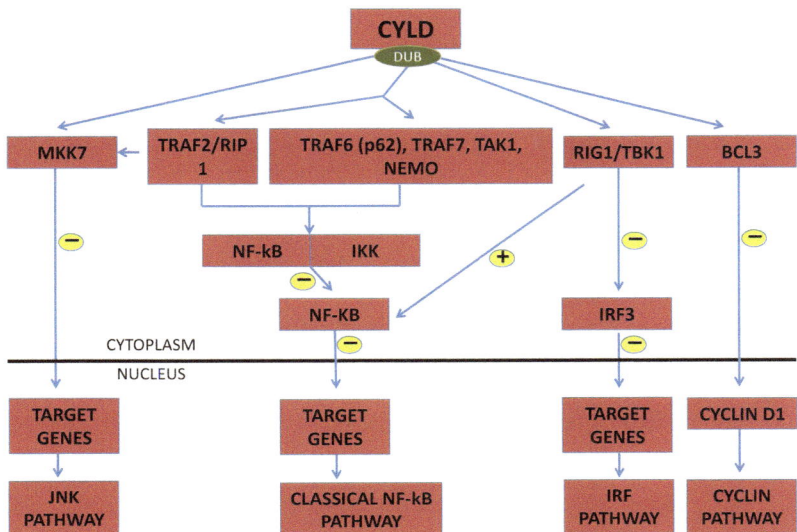

Fig. 4.5 Simplified schematic showing possible mechanisms of CYLD regulation of different signaling pathways of cell survival and proliferation through deubiquitination (*DUB*). *Arrows* denote multistep or incomplete pathways. CYLD deubiquitinates TRAF and its associated proteins RIP1, TRAF6 through the adaptor protein p62, TRAF7, TAK1, and NEMO, which inhibit downstream dissociation of NF-κB and IKK. CYLD-mediated deubiquitination of MKK7 and BCL-3 deactivates downstream JNK and cyclin D1 pathway, respectively. CYLD also negatively regulates IRF3 pathway by deubiquitination of RIG1 and TBK1

followed by c.2272C > T, c.2305delA, c.2172delA, and c.1112C > A. The overall *CYLD* mutation detection rate in BSS is 84 % (73/87) [86]. No correlation has been detected between *CYLD* mutations and a specific phenotype [86].

CYLD function has been reported primarily as a negative regulator of NF-κB signaling, a pathway shown to stimulate cell proliferation in a variety of tissues [87, 88] (Fig. 4.5). The NF-κB pathway is induced by a wide variety of stimuli including tumor necrosis factor-α (TNF-α) and interleukin-1 (IL-1). NF-κB suppression results in severe defects in the development of epidermal appendages, including hair follicles and sweat glands. However, the mechanism of aberrant NF-κB signaling and oncogenesis in the skin remains to be established. CYLD regulates the NF-κB pathway by deubiquitination of various targets; TRAF2 and its associated proteins; RIP1, TAK1, TRAF7, TRAF6 (occurs through a signal adaptor protein p62), and NEMO (NF-κB essential modulator). CYLD-mediated deubiquitination of target proteins subsequently inhibits downstream dissociation of IKK from NF-κB, leading to inhibition of the NF-κB pathway [89–95]. Loss of CYLD activity removes the inhibition of the NF-κB pathway, ultimately stimulating cell proliferation.

CYLD is also a negative regulator of JNK pathway, which plays a role in apoptosis, cell survival, and proliferation [96]. This regulation occurs in response to stimulation by several cytokines. Deubiquitination of TRAF2 by CYLD inhibits MKK7 activation and downstream JNK signaling [97, 98]. Also, CYLD deubiquitinates RIG-1/TBK1, which inhibits downstream activation of the growth promoting IRF3 signaling pathway [99, 100].

BCL-3 is a transcription factor that stimulates expression of cyclin D1. CYLD-mediated deubiquitination of BCL-3 prevents its translocation from the cytoplasm to the nucleus in response to UV light and subsequently inhibits the cyclin pathway, a cell cycle regulatory pathway. CYLD also affects cell proliferation and cycling by targeting Plk1 and histone deacetylase-6 (HDAC6) [101, 102]. It also has been shown to modulate cell migration via microtubule assembly and ion channel activity by deubiquitination of TRPA1 [103, 104].

The functions of *CYLD* still need further investigation, but there are multiple reports proposing *CYLD* as a tumor suppressor gene. Truncating mutations are found to be the most common tumor-predisposing germline mutations in *CYLD* (approximately 90 %). Most of the tumors show loss of heterozygosity (LOH) of the wild-type allele at the *CYLD* locus (chromosome 16q12–13) and some tumors without LOH have somatic mutations of *CYLD* [83, 85, 105–107]

Genetic Testing

CYLD mutation detection rate in BSS is relatively high, with 84 % of affected patients having mutations in the gene. Genetic testing for *CYLD* mutations, exons 16–20 in particular, is useful for identifying affected individuals as over 75 % of BSS families have a mutation in these regions [86]. In families with history of a severe phenotype and a confirmed *CYLD* mutation in a parent or sibling, prenatal testing for pregnancies should be performed [86]. Early identification of mutations and management of skin appendageal tumors can potentially minimize psychological burden due to disfigurement and promote early detection of malignant lesions. Further studies to identify positive and negative regulators of CYLD are necessary for a complete understanding of the mechanisms by which CYLD regulates tumorigenesis, as well as for the development of novel therapies for adnexal tumors.

Hidradenoma

Recent studies have shown that the t(11;19)(q21;p13) translocation seen in certain salivary gland tumors (such as mucoepidermoid carcinoma and Warthin's tumor) resulting in fusion of N-terminal CREB-binding domain of TORC1 to the Notch coactivator MAML2 was also identified in clear cell nodular hidradenoma. By RT-PCR analysis, TORC1–MAML2 fusion transcript was revealed, consisting of exon 1 of TORC1 fused to exons 2–5 of MAML2 [108].

Molecular Alterations in Cutaneous Adnexal Tumors with Sebaceous Origin

Clinical and Histologic Features of Sebaceous Neoplasms

There is a wide spectrum of sebaceous neoplasms ranging from hamartomatous to benign to malignant entities and their classification is often controversial. The hamartomatous, ectopic, and some benign sebaceous lesions, such as sebaceous hyperplasia, are almost exclusively sporadic and there is currently no description of their association with systemic syndromes. Therefore, considering the scope of our publication, we further describe sebaceous lesions that may potentially have this association.

Sebaceous adenomas are benign tumors derived from sebaceous glands that occur commonly on the head and neck region of older individuals as tan-yellow, small (less than 5 mm) papules. Histologically, they have a lobular, organoid growth pattern, are well-circumscribed, and often connected to epithelial surface. Sebaceous adenomas have an increased number of basaloid cells within the lobules: more than the normal two-cell layers but less than 50% of the entire lesion [109] (Fig. 4.6).

Sebaceomas (sebaceous epitheliomas) are usually larger lesions, typically ranging from 5 to 10 mm, are fleshy yellow and also occur in the head and neck region. Histologically, the sebaceomas have a lobular growth pattern, similar to sebaceous adenomas, but differ from them by the marked increased number of basaloid, germinative cells (more than 50% of the lesion), and lack the organoid pattern. Often sebaceomas involve dermis, but sometimes, connection with epidermal surface is noted. They are well-circumscribed lesions and there is no significant cytologic atypia or increased number of mitotic figures [110]. However, due to its higher proportion of basaloid, germinative cells and sometimes less obvious presence of mature sebocytes, sebaceomas may be difficult to distinguish from basal cell

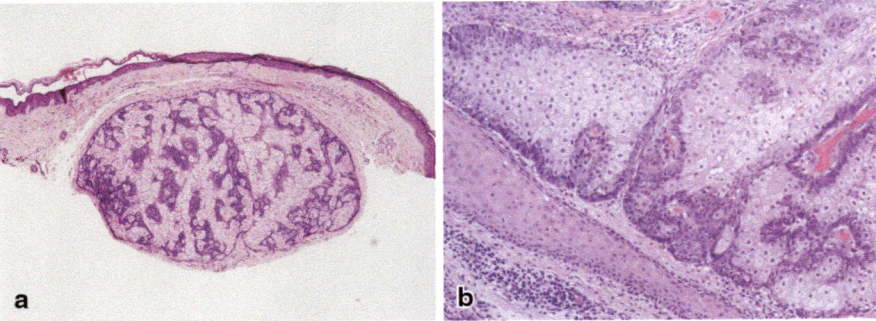

Fig. 4.6 Sebaceous adenoma—Histologically there is a well-circumscribed lobular, organoid growth pattern with an increased number of basaloid cells within the lobules (**a**), more than the normal two-cell layers but less than 50% of the entire lesion (**b**)

carcinomas. The lack of peripheral retraction artifact and associated myxoid stoma is helpful in the differential diagnosis.

Sebaceous carcinomas are relatively uncommon cutaneous malignant tumors. They may potentially develop from any sebaceous gland, approximately 75 % of cases occur on the eyelids (most common on the upper eyelid), arising mainly from meibomian glands of the tarsal plate and less commonly from the glands of Zeis [111–113]. Extraocular sebaceous carcinomas are predominately seen in the head and neck area, but can also arise on the trunk, extremities, vulva, penis, etc. [114, 115]. The distinction is of importance since it has been described that the two groups have different clinical course; the ocular sebaceous carcinomas have a lesser likelihood of association with Muir–Torre syndrome (see below) than their extraocular counterpart [116].

Although rare, sebaceous carcinoma is a malignancy with potentially aggressive behavior. Local recurrence complicates 6–29 % of periocular sebaceous cell carcinoma cases [117–121]. Regional or distal metastases affect 14–25 % of patients with a 5-year mortality ranging from 30 % (7–8) to 50–67 % according to different reports [117–121]. The prognosis of extraocular adnexal carcinoma is uncertain. Although it has been described that extraocular sebaceous carcinomas may give rise to regional metastases, it was originally thought that the mortality derived from these cases was low [114, 115, 122, 123]. However, more recently, it has been shown that these cases may have similar metastatic and fatality rates as their ocular counterparts [123].

Histologically, sebaceous carcinomas are characterized by an infiltrative growth pattern within the dermis and often, in the case of the periocular location, with an extension into the skeletal muscle and subcutaneous adipose tissue of the eyelid. The tumor cells have marked cytologic atypia and conspicuous mitotic figures, occasionally atypical. In well-differentiated tumors, the sebaceous differentiation is usually easily recognized, but in the poorly differentiated forms, mature sebocytes are not conspicuous and the diagnosis is often challenging. Pagetoid intraepithelial spread of neoplastic cells is a common feature and tumor necrosis is often noted (Fig. 4.7a, b).

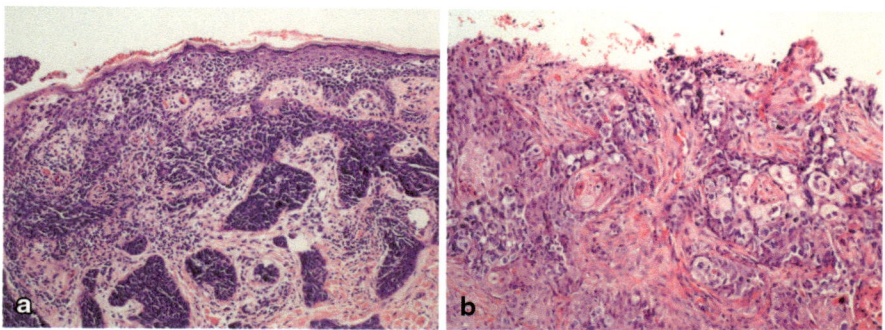

Fig. 4.7 Sebaceous carcinoma has infiltrative growth pattern within the dermis, the tumor cells have marked cytologic atypia and conspicuous mitotic figures, occasionally atypical (**a**). Pagetoid intraepithelial spread of neoplastic cells is a common feature and tumor necrosis is often noted (**b**)

Sebaceous tumors may occur de novo but their potential association with internal malignancies and Muir–Torre syndrome was increasingly recognized in the recent years and their distinction is of utmost clinical significance.

Muir–Torre Syndrome

Lynch syndrome or hereditary human nonpolyposis colorectal carcinoma (HNPCC) is an autosomal dominant inherited condition that predisposes individuals to develop frequently multiple, colorectal carcinoma and other malignancies, such as endometrial, ovarian, or gastric carcinomas at an early age. On clinical grounds alone, Lynch syndrome may be diagnosed based on "Amsterdam criteria" if: (1) three or more relatives, including at least one first-degree relative, are diagnosed with colorectal cancers; (2) colorectal cancers affect at least two generations; and (3) one or more cases of colorectal cancers are diagnosed before the age of 50 [124, 125]. Molecularly, Lynch syndrome is associated with germline mutations in DNA mismatch repair (MMR) genes *MLH1, MSH2, MSH6,* and *PMS2*. When a somatic loss-of-function alteration in the wild-type allele occurs, it leads to genomic microsatellite instability (MSI) [124–126].

Muir–Torre syndrome (MTS) is a phenotypic variant of Lynch syndrome, is identified in a small subset of patients with this condition, and is characterized by sebaceous neoplasms and less commonly keratoacathomas, either preceding or occurring concomitantly with internal malignancies [127–130]. The internal neoplasms commonly seen in Muir–Torre syndrome are colorectal carcinomas and genitourinary tract tumors, such as renal, bladder, ovarian, or endometrial carcinomas, and less commonly breast, hematologic, head and neck, or upper gastrointestinal tumors were reported. MTS was independently described in 1967 by Muir and Torre, and in 1981 Lynch suggested the relationship between HNPCC and MTS based on the observation that a subset of patients with HNPCC appeared to fulfill the criteria for MTS [127–130]. Interestingly, both cutaneous and visceral neoplasms in MTS patients have been shown to behave less aggressively compared with their sporadic counterparts.

MTS, similarly to HNPCC, often has defects and mutational inactivation of MMR genes. The role of the MMR genes is to remove errors made by DNA polymerase, such as mispairing of nucleotides during DNA replication, especially in regions of DNA (termed microsatellites) characterized by short mono- or dinuclotide repeats in elongation phase [131]. If MMR genes are inactivated, thus deficient, these errors accumulate and create MSI. The mismatch repair system is composed of human mutL homolog 1 (hMLH1), human mutS homolog 2 (hMSH2), human mutS homolog 6 (hMSH6), human mutS homolog 3 (hMSH3), human postmeiotic segregation increased 2 (hPMS2) proteins, among others. Initially a complex of hMSH2 and hMSH6 binds to erroneous DNA segment and then recruits hMLH1 and hPMS2 leading to excision of DNA segment [131–134]. MSI is caused by mutations occurring primarily on *MSH-2* or *MLH-1* MMR genes, which lead to reduction of corresponding proteins expression and are responsible for initial mis-match DNA recognition and triggering the repair process [127]. Mutations in *MSH1* and *MSH2* have the most severe effect producing high-grade microsatellite instabil-ity (h-MSI phenotype), frequently seen in HNPCC patients. MSI can be confirmed by polymerase chain reaction (PCR)-based analysis and chromatographic or elec-trophoretic assessment of multiple microsatellite lesions of DNA. In MTS, muta-tions of *MHS2* locus are more commonly seen (90 %) than *MLH1* gene mutations [127]. Most recently, lack of expression of *MSH6* in sebaceous lesions of MTS patients suggests that the *MSH6* gene mutation is also common and considering that *MSH6* forms a heterodimer with *MSH2*, it is understandable that mutations of *MSH2* lead to *MSH6* loss and is not necessary reflective of a germline mutation in *MSH6* [135]. Isolated mutations in *MSH6* are exceptionally noted but MTS is not definitely yet linked to isolated loss of MSH3 or PMS [135].

Sporadic sebaceous neoplasms do not show MSI and in these lesions *TP53* muta-tions have been recently reported, without a definite UV induction, and by immuno-histochemistry increased levels of p53 were described in carcinoma and not benign conditions [136, 137]. In addition, p21, an inhibitor of cyclin-dependent kinases induced by p53-dependent and independent pathways, correlates with higher rate of lymph node metastases [136, 138]. Even more recently, Wnt/β-catenin pathway and the downstream target lymphoid enhancer binding factor 1 (Lef-1) were described as having a role in the pathogenesis of sebaceous carcinomas [139]. Interestingly, it was reported that sebaceous neoplasms, including benign ones, have *LEF1* muta-tions irrespective of their DNA mismatch repair status. The mutations impair LEF1 binding to β-catenin and inactivate Wnt signaling [140, 141]. Mutations in the frag-ile histidine triad tumor suppressor gene, a suppressor of β-catenin transcriptional activity was recently described in sebaceous carcinoma, irrespective of their MSI status [142].

Genetic Testing and Clinical Follow-Up

In almost 40 % of MTS patients, a sebaceous neoplasm was the first clinical mani-festation of the syndrome and it was reported that as many as 63 % of the MTS pa-tients presenting with a sebaceous neoplasm have a concurrent internal malignancy or develop an additional one [143]. Therefore, early diagnosis of MTS is crucial not only for the patient but also may prompt familial genetic testing.

The gold standard for detecting MSI status of a patient is PCR analysis. How-ever, in the daily pathology practice, this testing is costly and not always available. A currently accepted method to evaluate for the functional status of MMR proteins within the sebaceous neoplasms is the use of immunohistochemistry using antibod-ies against MMR proteins, such as MLH1, MSH2, MSH6, and PMS1 [144–146].

The most common sebaceous neoplasm associated with MTS is sebaceous ad-enoma, but sebaceomas, sebaceous carcinomas, and occasionally keratoacanthomas are also seen in MTS patients. Certain histologic features and characteristics of se-baceous neoplasms that are more commonly associated with MTS are: (1) presence

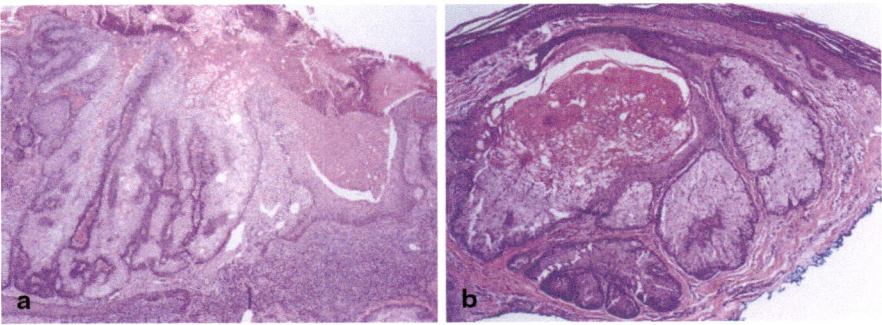

Fig. 4.8 Some of the sebaceous lesions associated with Muir–Torre syndrome were described as having characteristic appearance, such as keratoacanthoma-like architecture (**a**) or cystic appearance (**b**)

of multiple lesions, often outside of the head and neck area, (2) sebaceous carcinomas, especially extraocular, diagnosed at an early age, (3) sebaceous lesions with keratoacanthoma-like architecture or possible cystic changes (there is no definite agreement between the studies), and (4) presence of increased associated lymphocytic infiltrate has been shown to correlate with MSI, similar to MSI-associated HNPCC [147, 148] (Fig. 4.8a, b).

Immunohistochemical studies can be used to reveal loss of one or more MMR proteins in sebaceous neoplasms in MTS patients and are reported to have a relatively good sensitivity and specificity (Fig. 4.9a, b, c). Staining from these proteins is nuclear and is interpreted as loss of expression in comparison with the internal control (epidermis, non-lesional sebaceous cells). It has been reported that in patients with MTS, 55–86 % of sebaceous adenomas have loss of MSH2, 31–100 % in sebaceous carcinoma, and only 17 % in sebaceomas. MSH6 is reported being lost in 50–78 % of sebaceous adenomas, 33 % in sebaceomas, and 100 % in sebaceous carcinoma. Absence of MLH1 varies between 14 and 33 % of sebaceous adenomas, 83 % in sebaceoma, and 31 % in sebaceous carcinomas. In studies using unselected sebaceous neoplasms, the positive predictive value for MTS is reported as 33–88 % for MLH1, 55–66 % for MSH2, and 67 % for MSH6 [144–146].

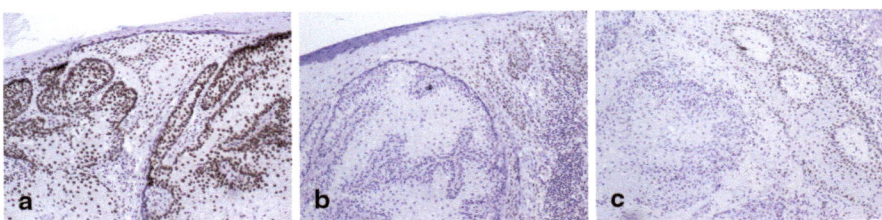

Fig. 4.9 Immunohistochemical studies for MLH1 (**a**), MSH2 (**b**), and MSH6 (**c**) in a patient with Muir–Torre syndrome reveal preservation of MLH1 (**a**), loss of MSH2 (**b**), and MSH6 (**c**)

References

1. Chan P, White SW, Pierson DL, Rodman OG. Trichilemmoma. J Dermatol Surg Oncol. 1979;5(1):58–9.
2. Hidayat AA, Font RL. Trichilemmoma of eyelid and eyebrow: a clinicopathologic study of 31 cases. Arch Ophthalmol. 1980;98(5):844–7.
3. Lloyd KM 2nd, Dennis M. Cowden's disease. A possible new symptom complex with multiple system involvement. Ann Intern Med. 1963;58:136–42.
4. Eng C. Will the real Cowden syndrome please stand up: revised diagnostic criteria. J Med Genet. 2000;37(11):828–30.
5. Salem OS, Steck WD. Cowden's disease (multiple hamartoma and neoplasia syndrome): a case report and review of the English literature. J Am Acad Dermatol. 1983;8(5):686–96.
6. Starink TM, Meijer CJ, Brownstein MH. The cutaneous pathology of Cowden's disease: new findings. J Cutan Pathol. 1985;12(2):83–93.
7. Starink TM, Hausman R. The cutaneous pathology of facial lesions in Cowden's disease. J Cutan Pathol. 1984;11(5):331–37
8. Brownstein MH, Mehregan AH, Bikowski JB, Lupulescu A, Patterson JC. The dermatopathology of Cowden's syndrome. Br J Dermatol. 1979;100(6):667–73.
9. Starink TM, van der Veen JP, Arwert F, et al. The Cowden syndrome: a clinical and genetic study in 21 patients. Clin Genet. 1986;29(3):222–33.
10. Harach HR, Soubeyran I, Brown A, Bonneau D, Longy M. Thyroid pathologic findings in patients with Cowden disease. Ann Diagn Pathol. 1999;3:331–40.
11. Schrager CA, Schneider D, Gruener AC, Tsou HC, Peacocke M. Clinical and pathological features of breast disease in Cowden's syndrome: an underrecognized syndrome with an increased risk of breast cancer. Hum Pathol. 1998;29:47–53.
12. Brownstein MH, Wolf M, Bikowski JB. Cowden's disease: a cutaneous marker of breast cancer. Cancer. 1978;41(6):2393–8.
13. Tan WH, Baris HN, Burrows PE, et al. The spectrum of vascular anomalies in patients with PTEN mutations: implications for diagnosis and management. J Med Genet. 2007;44:594–602.
14. Fistarol SK, Anliker MD, Itin PH. Cowden disease or multiple hamartoma syndrome—cutaneous clue to internal malignancy. Eur J Dermatol. 2002;12(5):411–21.
15. Tan MH, Mester JL, Ngeow J, Rybicki LA, Orloff MS, Eng C. Lifetime cancer risks in individuals with germline PTEN mutations. Clin Cancer Res. 2012;18(2):400–7.
16. Nusbaum R, Vogel KJ, Ready K. Susceptibility to breast cancer: hereditary syndromes and low penetrance genes. Breast Dis. 2006;27:21–50.
17. Blumenthal GM, Dennis PA. PTEN hamartoma tumor syndromes. Eur J Hum Genet. 2008;16(11):1289–300.
18. Nelen MR, Padberg GW, Peeters EA, et al. Localization of the gene for Cowden disease to chromosome 10q22-23. Nat Genet. 1996;13(1):114–6.
19. Li J, Yen C, Liaw D, et al. PTEN, a putative protein tyrosine phosphatase gene mutated in human brain, breast, and prostate cancer. Science. 1997;275(5308):1943–7.
20. Liaw D, Marsh DJ, Li J, et al. Germline mutations of the PTEN gene in Cowden disease, an inherited breast and thyroid cancer syndrome. Nat Genet. 1997;16(1):64–7.
21. Eng C. PTEN: one gene, many syndromes. Hum Mutat. 2003;22(3):183–98.
22. Hobert JA, Eng C. PTEN hamartoma tumor syndrome: an overview. Genet Med. 2009;11(10):687–94.
23. Zhou XP, Waite KA, Pilarski R, et al. Germline PTEN promoter mutations and deletions in Cowden/Bannayan–Riley–Ruvalcaba syndrome result in aberrant PTEN protein and dysregulation of the phosphoinositol–3–kinase/Akt pathway. Am J Hum Genet. 2003;73(2):404–11.
24. Marsh DJ, Coulon V, Lunetta KL, et al. Mutation spectrum and genotype–phenotype analyses in Cowden disease and Bannayan–Zonana syndrome, two hamartoma syndromes with germline PTEN mutation. Hum Mol Genet. 1998;7(3):507–15.
25. Trotman LC, Wang X, Alimonti A, et al. Ubiquitination regulates PTEN nuclear import and tumor suppression. Cell. 2007;128(1):141–56.
26. Orloff MS, He X, Peterson C, et al. Germline PIK3CA and AKT1 mutations in Cowden and Cowden-like syndromes. Am J Hum Genet. 2013;92(1):76–80.

27. Cho YJ, Liang P. Killin is a p53-regulated nuclear inhibitor of DNA synthesis. Proc Natl Acad Sci U S A. 2008;105(14):5396–401.
28. Bennett KL, Mester J, Eng C. Germline epigenetic regulation of KILLIN in Cowden and Cowden-like syndrome. JAMA. 2010;304(24):2724–31.
29. Al-Zaid T, Ditelberg JS, Prieto VG, et al. Trichilemmomas show loss of PTEN in Cowden syndrome but only rarely in sporadic tumors. J Cutan Pathol. 2012;39(5):493–9.
30. Julian CG, Bowers PW. A clinical review of 209 pilomatricomas. J Am Acad Dermatol. 1998;39(2, pt 1):191–95.
31. Lan MY, Lan MC, Ho CY, Li WY, Lin CZ. Pilomatricoma of the head and neck: a retrospective review of 179 cases. Arch Otolaryngol Head Neck Surg. 2003;129(12):1327–30.
32. Marrogi AJ, Wick MR, Dehner LP. Pilomatrical neoplasms in children and young adults. Am J Dermatopathol. 1992;14(2):87–94.
33. O'Connor N, Patel M, Umar T, Macpherson DW, Ethunandan M. Head and neck pilomatricoma: an analysis of 201 cases. Br J Oral Maxillofac Surg. 2011;49(5):354–8.
34. Berberian BJ, Colonna TM, Battaglia M, Sulica VI. Multiple pilomatricomas in association with myotonic dystrophy and a family history of melanoma. J Am Acad Dermatol. 1997;37(2, pt 1):268–69.
35. Cambiaghi S, Ermacora E, Brusasco A, Canzi L, Caputo R. Multiple pilomatricomas in Rubinstein–Taybi syndrome: a case report. Pediatr Dermatol. 1994;11(1):21–5.
36. Cooper PH, Fechner RE. Pilomatricoma-like changes in the epidermal cysts of Gardner's syndrome. J Am Acad Dermatol. 1983;8(5):639–44.
37. Wood S, Nguyen D, Hutton K, Dickson W. Pilomatricomas in Turner syndrome. Pediatr Dermatol. 2008;25(4):449–51.
38. Chan EF, Gat U, McNiff JM, Fuchs E. A common human skin tumour is caused by activating mutations in beta-catenin. Nat Genet. 1999;21(4):410–3.
39. Kajino Y, Yamaguchi A, Hashimoto N, Matsuura A, Sato N, Kikuchi K. beta-Catenin gene mutation in human hair follicle-related tumors. Pathol Int. 2001;51(7):543–8.
40. Moon RT, Kohn AD, De Ferrari GV, Kaykas A. WNT and beta-catenin signalling: diseases and therapies. Nat Rev Genet. 2004;5(9):691–701.
41. van Es JH, Barker N, Clevers H. You Wnt some, you lose some: oncogenes in the Wnt signaling pathway. Curr Opin Genet Dev. 2003;13(1):28–33.
42. Clevers H. Wnt/beta-catenin signaling in development and disease. Cell. 2006;127(3):469–80.
43. Moreno-Bueno G, Gamallo C, Perez-Gallego L, Contreras F, Palacios J. beta-catenin expression in pilomatrixomas: relationship with beta-catenin gene mutations and comparison with beta-catenin expression in normal hair follicles. Br J Dermatol. 2001;145(4):576–81.
44. Behrens J, von Kries JP, Kuhl M, et al. Functional interaction of beta-catenin with the transcription factor LEF-1. Nature. 1996;382(6592):638–42.
45. MacDonald BT, Tamai K, He X. Wnt/beta-catenin signaling: components, mechanisms, and diseases. Dev Cell. 2009;17(1):9–26.
46. Farrier S, Morgan M. bcl-2 expression in pilomatricoma. Am J Dermatopathol. 1997; 19(3):254–7.
47. Toro JR, Wei M-H, Glenn GM, et al. BHD mutations, clinical and molecular genetic investigations of Birt–Hogg–Dube syndrome: a new series of 50 families and a review of published reports. J Med Genet. 2008;45(6):321–31.
48. Toro JR, Glenn G, Duray P, Darling T, Weirich G, Zbar B, Linehan M, Turner ML. Birt–Hogg–Dubé syndrome: a novel marker of kidney neoplasia. Arch Dermatol. 1999;135(10):1195–202.
49. Birt AR, Hogg GR, Dube WJ. Hereditary multiple fibrofolliculomas with trichodiscomas and acrochordons. Arch Dermatol. 1977;113(12):1674–7.
50. Gijezen LM, Vernooij M, Martens H, et al. Topical rapamycin as a treatment for fibrofolliculomas in Birt–Hogg–Dubé syndrome: a double-blind placebo-controlled randomized split-face trial. PLoS ONE. 2014;9(6):e99071.
51. Schmidt LS, Warren MB, Nickerson ML, et al. Birt–Hogg–Dubé syndrome, a genodermatosis associated with spontaneous pneumothorax and kidney neoplasia, maps to chromosome 17p11.2. Am J Hum Genet. 2001;69:876–82.
52. Fujita WH, Barr RJ, Headley JL. Multiple fibrofolliculomas with trichodiscomas and acrochordons. Arch Dermatol. 1981;117:32–5.

53. Misago N, Kimura T, Narisawa Y. Fibrofolliculoma/trichodiscoma and fibrous papule (peri-follicular fibroma/angiofibroma): a revaluation of the histopathological and immunohisto-chemical features. J Cutan Pathol. 2009;36(9):943–51.

54. Murakami Y, Wataya-Kaneda M, Tanaka M, et al. Two Japanese cases of Birt–Hogg–Dubé syndrome with pulmonary cysts, fibrofolliculomas, and renal cell carcinomas. Case Rep Dermatol. 2014;6(1):20–8.

55. Zbar B, Alvord WG, Glenn G, et al. Risk of renal and colonic neoplasms and spontaneous pneumothorax in the Birt–Hogg–Dube syndrome. Cancer Epidemiol Biomarkers Prev. 2002;11:393–400.

56. Khoo SK, Bradley M, Wong FK, et al. Birt–Hogg–Dube syndrome: mapping of a novel hereditary neoplasia gene to chromosome 17p12–q11.2. Oncogene. 2001;20:5239–42.

57. Schmidt LS, Nickerson ML, Warren MB, et al. Germline BHD-mutation spectrum and phenotype analysis of a large cohort of families with Birt–Hogg–Dubé syndrome. Am J Hum Genet. 2005;76(6):1023–33.

58. Nickerson ML, Warren MB, Toro JR, et al. Mutations in a novel gene lead to kidney tumors, lung wall defects, and benign tumors of the hair follicle in patients with the Birt–Hogg–Dubé syndrome. Cancer Cell. 2002;2(2):157–64.

59. Vocke CD, Yang Y, Pavlovich CP, et al. High frequency of somatic frameshift BHD gene mutations in Birt–Hogg–Dubé-associated renal tumors. J Natl Cancer Inst. 2005;97(12):931–5.

60. van Steensel MA, Verstraeten VL, Frank J, et al. Novel mutations in the BHD gene and absence of loss of heterozygosity in fibrofolliculomas of Birt–Hogg–Dubé patients. J Invest Dermatol. 2007;127(3):588–93.

61. Baba M, Hong SB, Sharma N, et al. Folliculin encoded by the BHD gene interacts with a binding protein, FNIP1, and AMPK, and is involved in AMPK and mTOR signaling. Proc Natl Acad Sci U S A. 2006;103(42):15552–7.

62. Hasumi H, Baba M, Hong SB, et al. Identification and characterization of a novel folliculin-interacting protein FNIP2. Gene. 2008;415(1–2):60–7.

63. Hong SB, Oh H, Valera VA, et al. Inactivation of the FLCN tumor suppressor gene induces TFE3 transcriptional activity by increasing its nuclear localization. PLoS ONE. 2010;5(12):e15793.

64. Singh SR, Zhen W, Zheng Z, et al. The Drosophila homolog of the human tumor suppressor gene BHD interacts with the JAK-STAT and Dpp signaling pathways in regulating male germline stem cell maintenance. Oncogene. 2006;25(44):5933–41.

65. Lim DH, Rehal PK, Nahorski MS, et al. A new locus-specific database (LSDB) for mutations in the folliculin (FLCN) gene. Hum Mutat. 2010;31(1):E1043–51.

66. Wei MH, Blake PW, Shevchenko J, et al. The folliculin mutation database: an online database of mutations associated with Birt–Hogg–Dubé syndrome. Hum Mutat. 2009;30(9):E880–90.

67. Menko FH, van Steensel MA, Giraud S, et al. Birt–Hogg–Dubé syndrome: diagnosis and management. Lancet Oncol. 2009;10(12):1199–206.

68. Lee DA, Grossman ME, Schneiderman P, et al. Genetics of skin appendage neoplasms and related syndromes. J Med Genet. 2005;42(11):811–9.

69. Welch J, Wells R, Kerr C. Ancell–Spiegler Cylindromas (turban tumors) and Brooke–Fordyce Trichoepitheliomas: evidence for a single genetic entity. J Med Genet. 1968;5:29–35.

70. Ancell H. History of a remarkable case of tumours developed on the head and face; accompanied with a similar disease in the abdomen. Med Chir Trans. 1842;25:227–46.

71. Spiegler E. Ueber Endoteliome der Haut. AMA Arch Dermatol Syphilis. 1899;50:163–76.

72. Brooke H. Epithelioma adenoides cysticum. Br J Dermatol Syphilis. 1892;4:286–96.

73. Fordyce J. Multiple benign cystic epithelioma of the skin. J Cutan Dis. 1892;10:459–73.

74. Gottschalk HR. Proceedings: dermal eccrine cylindroma, epithelioma adenoides cysticum of Brooke, and eccrine spiradenoma. Arch Dermatol. 1974;110:473–4.

75. Bumgardner AC, Hsu S, Nunez-Gussman JK, Schwartz MR. Trichoepitheliomas and eccrine spiradenomas with spiradenoma/cylindroma overlap. Int J Dermatol. 2005;44(5):415–7.

76. Burrows NP, Jones RR, Smith NP. The clinicopathological features of familial cylindromas and trichoepitheliomas (Brooke-Spiegler syndrome): a report of two families. Clin Exp Dermatol. 1992;17:332–6.

77. Kazakov DV, Zelger B, Rutten A, et al. Morphologic diversity of malignant neoplasms arising in preexisting spiradenoma, cylindroma, and spiradenocylindroma based on the study of 24 cases, sporadic or occurring in the setting of Brooke-Spiegler syndrome. Am J Surg Pathol. 2009;33(5):705–19.
78. Harada H, Hashimoto K, Ko MS. The gene for multiple familial trichoepithelioma maps to chromosome 9p21. J Invest Dermatol. 1996;107:41–3.
79. Uede K, Yamamoto Y, Furukawa F. Brooke-Spiegler syndrome associated with cylindroma, trichoepithelioma, spiradenoma, and syringoma. J Dermatol. 2004;31(1):32–8.
80. Lian F, Cockerell CJ. Cutaneous appendage tumors: familial cylindromatosis and associated tumors update. Adv Dermatol. 2005;21:217–34.
81. Alsaad KO, Obaidat NA, Ghazarian D. Skin adnexal neoplasms—part 1: an approach to tumours of the pilosebaceous unit. J Clin Pathol. 2007;60(2):129–44.
82. Obaidat NA, Alsaad KO, Ghazarian D. Skin adnexal neoplasms—part 2: an approach to tumours of cutaneous sweat glands. J Clin Pathol. 2007;60(2):145–59.
83. Biggs PJ, Wooster R, Ford D, Chapman P, Mangion J, Quirk Y, Easton DF, Burn J, Stratton MR. Familial cylindromatosis (turban tumour syndrome) gene localised to chromosome 16q12–q13: evidence for its role as a tumour suppressor gene. Nat Genet. 1995;11:441–3.
84. Takahashi M, Rapley E, Biggs PJ, Lakhani SR, Cooke D, Hansen J, Blair E, Hofmann B, Siebert R, Turner G, Evans DG, Schrander-Stumpel C, Beemer FA, van Vloten WA, Breuning MH, van den Ouweland A, Halley D, Delpech B, Cleveland M, Leigh I, Chapman P, Burn J, Hohl D, Gorog JP, Seal S, Mangion J. Linkage and LOH studies in 19 cylindromatosis families show no evidence of genetic heterogeneity and refine the CYLD locus on chromosome 16q12–q13. Hum Genet. 2000;106:58–65.
85. Bignell GR, Warren W, Seal S, Takahashi M, Rapley E, Barfoot R, Green H, Brown C, Biggs PJ, Lakhani SR, Jones C, Hansen J, Blair E, Hofmann B, Siebert R, Turner G, Evans DG, Schrander- Stumpel C, Beemer FA, van Den Ouweland A, Halley D, Delpech B, Cleveland MG, Leigh I, Leisti J, Rasmussen S. Identification of the familial cylindromatosis tumour-suppressor gene. Nat Genet. 2000;25:160–5.
86. Black PW, Toro JR. Update of cylindromatosis gene (CYLD) mutations in Brooke–Spiegler syndrome: novel insights into the role of deubiquitination in cell signaling. Hum Mutat. 2009;30(7):1025–36.
87. Karin M, Cao Y, Greten FR, Li ZW. NF-κB in cancer: from innocent bystander to major culprit. Nat Rev Cancer. 2002;2:301–10.
88. Perkins ND. Integrating cell-signalling pathways with NF-κB and IKK function. Nat Rev Mol Cell Biol. 2007;8:49–62.
89. Hacker H, Karin M Regulation and function of IKK and IKK-related kinases. Sci STKE. 2006;2006:re13.
90. Brummelkamp TR, Nijman SM, Dirac AM, Bernards R. Loss of the cylindromatosis tumour suppressor inhibits apoptosis by activating NF-κB. Nature. 2003;424:797–801.
91. Kovalenko A, Chable-Bessia C, Cantarella G, Israel A, Wallach D, Courtois G. The tumour suppressor CYLD negatively regulates NF-κB signalling by deubiquitination. Nature. 2003;424:801–5.
92. Trompouki E, Hatzivassiliou E, Tsichritzis T, Farmer H, Ashworth A, Mosialos G. CYLD is a deubiquitinating enzyme that negatively regulates NF-κB activation by TNFR family members. Nature. 2003;424:793–6.
93. Reiley WW, Jin W, Lee AJ, Wright A, Wu X, Tewalt EF, Leonard TO, Norbury CC, Fitzpatrick L, Zhang M, Sun SC. Deubiquitinating enzyme CYLD negatively regulates the ubiquitin-dependent kinase Tak1 and prevents abnormal T cell responses. J Exp Med. 2007;204:1475–85.
94. Wooten MW, Geetha T, Babu JR, Seibenhener ML, Peng J, Cox N, Diaz-Meco MT, Moscat J. Essential role of sequestosome 1/p62 in regulating accumulation of Lys63-ubiquitinated proteins. J Biol Chem. 2008;283:6783–9.
95. Regamey A, Hohl D, Liu JW, Roger T, Kogerman P, Toftgard R, Huber M. The tumor suppressor CYLD interacts with TRIP and regulates negatively nuclear factor κB activation by tumor necrosis factor. J Exp Med. 2003;198:1959–64.

96. Reiley W, Zhang M, Sun SC. Negative regulation of JNK signaling by the tumor suppressor CYLD. J Biol Chem. 2004;279:55161–7.
97. Xue L, Igaki T, Kuranaga E, Kanda H, Miura M, Xu T. Tumor suppressor CYLD regulates JNK-induced cell death in drosophila. Dev Cell. 2007;13:446–54.
98. Koga T, Lim JH, Jono H, Ha UH, Xu H, Ishinaga H, Morino S, Xu X, Yan C, Kai H, Li JD. Tumor suppressor cylindromatosis acts as a negative regulator for streptococcus pneumoniae-induced NFAT signaling. J Biol Chem. 2008;283:12546–54.
99. Friedman CS, O'Donnell MA, Legarda-Addison D, Ng A, Cardenas WB, Yount JS, Moran TM, Basler CF, Komuro A, Horvath CM, Xavier R, Ting AT. The tumour suppressor CYLD is a negative regulator of RIG-I-mediated antiviral response. EMBO Rep. 2008;9:930–6.
100. Zhang M, Wu X, Lee AJ, Jin W, Chang M, Wright A, Imaizumi T, Sun SC. Regulation of IκB kinase-related kinases and antiviral responses by tumor suppressor CYLD. J Biol Chem. 2008;283:18621–6.
101. Stegmeier F, Sowa ME, Nalepa G, Gygi SP, Harper JW, Elledge SJ. The tumor suppressor CYLD regulates entry into mitosis. Proc Natl Acad Sci U S A. 2007;104:8869–74.
102. Wickström SA, Masoumi KC, Khochbin S, Fässler R, Massoumi R. CYLD negatively regulates cell-cycle progression by inactivating HDAC6 and increasing the levels of acetylated tubulin. EMBO J. 2010;29(1):131–44.
103. Gao J, Huo L, Sun X, Liu M, Li D, Dong JT, Zhou J. The tumor suppressor CYLD regulates microtubule dynamics and plays a role in cell migration. J Biol Chem. 2008;283:8802–9.
104. Stokes A, Wakano C, Koblan-Huberson M, Adra CN, Fleig A, Turner H. TRPA1 is a substrate for de- ubiquitination by the tumor suppressor CYLD. Cell Signal. 2006;18:1584–94.
105. Leonard N, Chaggar R, Jones C, Takahashi M, Nikitopoulou A, Lakhani SR. Loss of heterozygosity at cylindromatosis gene locus, CYLD, in sporadic skin adnexal tumours. J Clin Pathol. 2001;54:689–92.
106. Thomson SA, Rasmussen SA, Zhang J, Wallace MR. A new hereditary cylindromatosis family associated with CYLD1 on chromosome 16. Hum Genet. 1999;105:171–3.
107. Massoumi R, Chmielarska K, Hennecke K, Pfeifer A, Fassler R. Cyld inhibits tumor cell proliferation by blocking bcl-3-dependent NF-kappaB signaling. Cell. 2006;125(4):665–77.
108. Behboudi A, Winnes M, Gorunova L, et al. Clear cell hidradenoma of the skin—a third tumor type with a t(11;19)-associated TORC1-MAML2 gene fusion. Genes Chromosomes Cancer. 2005;43(2):202–5.
109. Rulon DB, Helwig EB. Cutaneous sebaceous neoplasms. Cancer. 1974;33:82–102.
110. Misago N, Mihara I, Ansai S, Narisawa Y. Sebaceoma and related neoplasms with sebaceous differentiation: a clinicopathologic study of 30 cases. Am J Dermatopathol. 2002;24:294–304.
111. Song A, Carter KD, Syed NA, Song J, Nerad JA. Sebaceous cell carcinoma of the ocular adnexa: clinical presentations, histopathology, and outcomes. Ophthal Plast Reconstr Surg. 2008;24:194–200.
112. Nelson BR, Hamlet KR, Gillard BAM, et al. Sebaceous carcinoma. J Am Acad Dermatology. 1995;33:1.
113. Graham RM, McKee H, McGibbon D. Sebaceous carcinoma, Clin Exp Dermatol 1984;9:466.
114. Pricolo VE, Rodil JV, Vezeridis MP. Extraorbital sebaceous carcinoma. J Am Acad Dermatol. 1995;33:1.
115. Wick MR, Goellner JR, Wolfe JT, Su WPD. Adnexal carcinomas of the skin. II. Extraocular sebaceous carcinomas. Cancer. 1985;56:1163.
116. Singh RS, Grayson W, Redston M, et al. Site and tumor type predicts DNA mismatch repair status in cutaneous sebaceous neoplasia. Am J Surg Pathol. 2008;32:936–42.
117. Harvey JT, Anderson RL. The management of meibomian gland carcinoma. Ophthalmic Surg. 1982;13(1):56.
118. Rao NA, McLean IW, Zimmerman LE. Sebaceous carcinoma of the eyelid and caruncle: correlation of the clinical pathologic features with prognosis. In: Jakobiec FA, editor. Ocular and adnexal tumors. Birmingham: Aesculapius; 1978, p. 461.

119. Wolfe JT 3rd, Yeatts RP, Wick MR, Campbell RJ, Waller RR. Sebaceous carcinoma of the eyelid. Errors in clinical and pathologic diagnosis. Am J Surg Pathol. 1984;8(8):597.
120. Shields JA, Demirci H, Marr BP, Eagle RC Jr, Shields CL. Sebaceous carcinoma of the eyelids: personal experience with 60 cases. Ophthalmology. 2004;111(12):2151.
121. Rao NA, Hidayat AA, McLean IW, Zimmerman LE. Sebaceous carcinomas of the ocular adnexa: a clinicopathologic study of 104 cases, with five-year follow-up data. Hum Pathol. 1982;13:113.
122. Hernandez-Perez E, Banos E. Sebaceous carcinoma: report of two cases with metastasis. Dermatologica. 1978;156:184.
123. Moreno C, Jacyk WK, Judd MJ, et al. Highly aggressive extraocular sebaceous carcinoma. Am J Dermatopathol. 2001;23:450.
124. Abdel-Rahman WM, Peltomaki P. Lynch syndrome and related familial colorectal cancers. Crit Rev Oncog. 2008;14:1–22. Discussion 23–31.
125. Lynch HT1, Smyrk T. Hereditary nonpolyposis colorectal cancer (Lynch syndrome). An updated review. Cancer. 1996;78(6):1149–67.
126. Yuen ST, Chan TL, Ho JW, et al. Germline, somatic and epigenetic events underlying mismatch repair deficiency in colorectal and HNPCC-related cancers. Oncogene. 2002;21:7585–92.
127. Shalin SC, Lyle S, Calonje E, Lazar AJL. Sebaceous neoplasia and the Muir–Torre syndrome: important connections with clinical implications. Histopathology. 2010;56(1):133–47.
128. Dores GM, Curtis RE, Toro JR, Devesa SS, Fraumeni JF Jr. Incidence of cutaneous sebaceous carcinoma and risk of associated neoplasms: insight into Muir–Torre syndrome. Cancer. 2008;113:3372–81.
129. Schwartz RA, Torre DP. The Muir–Torre syndrome: a 25-year retrospect. J Am Acad Dermatol. 1995;33:90–104.
130. Cohen PR, Kohn SR, Davis DA, Kurzrock R. Muir–Torre syndrome. Dermatol Clin. 1995;13:79–89.
131. Entius MM, Keller JJ, Drillenburg P, Kuypers KC, Giardiello FM, Offerhaus GJ. Microsatellite instability and expression of hMLH-1 and hMSH-2 in sebaceous gland carcinomas as markers for Muir–Torre syndrome. Clin Cancer Res. 2000;6(5):1784–9.
132. Mathiak M, Rutten A, Mangold E, et al. Loss of DNA mismatch repair proteins in skin tumors from patients with Muir–Torre syndrome and MSH2 or MLH1 germline mutations: establishment of immunohistochemical analysis as a screening test. Am J Surg Pathol. 2002;26(3):338–43.
133. Kruse R, Ruzicka T. DNA mismatch repair and the significance of a sebaceous skin tumor for visceral cancer prevention. Trends Mol Med. 2004;10:136–41.
134. Mangold E, Pagenstecher C, Leister M, et al. A genotype–phenotype correlation in HNPCC: strong predominance of msh2 mutations in 41 patients with Muir–Torre syndrome. J Med Genet. 2004;41:567–72.
135. Chhibber V, Dresser K, Mahalingam M. MSH-6: extending the reliability of immunohistochemistry as a screening tool in Muir–Torre syndrome. Mod Pathol. 2008;21:159–64.
136. Kiyosaki K, Nakada C, Hijiya N, et al. Analysis of p53 mutations and the expression of p53 and p21WAF1/CIP1 protein in 15 cases of sebaceous carcinoma of the eyelid. Invest Ophthalmol Vis Sci. 2010;51(1):7–11.
137. Gonzalez-Fernandez F, Kaltreider SA, Patnaik BD, et al. Sebaceous carcinoma. Tumor progression through mutational inactivation of p53. Ophthalmology. 1998;105:497–506.
138. McBride SR, Leonard N, Reynolds NJ. Loss of p21(WAF1) compartmentalisation in sebaceous carcinoma compared with sebaceous hyperplasia and sebaceous adenoma. J Clin Pathol. 2002;55(10):763–6.
139. Niemann C, Owens DM, Hulsken J, Birchmeier W, Watt FM. Expression of DeltaNLef1 in mouse epidermis results in differentiation of hair follicles into squamous epidermal cysts and formation of skin tumours. Development. 2002;129:95–109.
140. Niemann C, Owens DM, Schettina P, Watt FM. Dual role of inactivating Lef1 mutations in epidermis: tumor promotion and specification of tumor type. Cancer Res. 2007;67:2916–21.

141. Takeda H, Lyle S, Lazar AJ, Zouboulis CC, Smyth I, Watt FM. Human sebaceous tumors harbor inactivating mutations in LEF1. Nat Med. 2006;12:395–7.
142. Zanesi N, Croce CM. Fragile histidine triad gene and skin cancer. Eur J Dermatol. 2001;11:401–4.
143. Jones B, Oh C, Mangold E, Egan CA. Muir–Torre syndrome: diagnostic and screening guidelines. Australas J Dermatol. 2006;47:266–9.
144. Orta L, Klimstra DS, Qin J, et al. Towards identification of hereditary DNA mismatch repair deficiency: sebaceous neoplasm warrants routine immunohistochemical screening regardless of patient's age or other clinical characteristics. Am J Surg Pathol. 2009;33:934–44.
145. Abbas O, Mahalingam M. Cutaneous sebaceous neoplasms as markers of Muir–Torre syndrome: a diagnostic algorithm. J Cutan Pathol. 2009;36:613–9.
146. Marcus VA, Madlensky L, Gryfe R, et al. Immunohistochemistry for hMLH1 and hMSH2: a practical test for DNA mismatch repair-deficient tumors. Am J Surg Pathol. 1999;23:1248–55.
147. Rutten A, Burgdorf W, Hugel H, et al. Cystic sebaceous tumors as marker lesions for the Muir–Torre syndrome: a histopathologic and molecular genetic study. Am J Dermatopathol. 1999;21:405–13.
148. Abbott JJ, Hernandez-Rios P, Amirkhan RH, Hoang MP. Cystic sebaceous neoplasms in Muir–Torre syndrome. Arch Pathol Lab Med. 2003;127:614–7.

Chapter 5
Infectious Diseases of the Skin

Carlos A. Torres-Cabala, Kudakwashe Mutyambizi and Francisco Bravo

Introduction

Traditional methods for detection of infectious agents affecting the skin are still widely used in the daily dermatopathology practice. Examination of histological sections stained with hematoxylin and eosin (H&E) and histochemical methods (e.g., Gram, periodic acid Schiff stain (PAS), Gomori's Methenamine Silver GMS, and acid-fast stains) remain as the initial and probably the definitive step in a high number of cases in which the diagnosis of an infectious disease of the skin is made. The value of these methodologies relies on their easy accessibility by the regular pathology laboratories. These traditional tests allow the dermatopathologists to identify or confirm the presence of an infectious microorganism within the skin sample; specific classification of the organism is usually very limited in these morphology-based techniques. Immunohistochemistry, utilizing specific antibodies against infectious microorganisms, is of great utility in certain cases of viral (e.g., Herpes virus), bacterial (e.g., *Treponema*), and fungal (e.g., dermatophytes) [1] infections. Besides the relatively long time that passes before a culture is positive, the fact that many microorganisms do not grow under certain conditions makes culture-based methods limited in specific clinical circumstances. Still, culture-based methods are regarded as the gold standard for the specific diagnosis of most of the infectious diseases of the skin.

There are some particularities that make molecular tests especially attractive for the infectious dermatopathology laboratory. These methods are highly sensitive

C. A. Torres-Cabala (✉)
Departments of Pathology and Dermatology, The University of Texas: MD Anderson Cancer Center, 1515 Holcombe Blvd, Unit 85, Houston, TX 77030, USA
e-mail: ctcabala@mdanderson.org

K. Mutyambizi
Department of Pathology and Dermatology, University of Texas: MD Anderson Cancer Center, Houston, TX, USA

F. Bravo
Departments of Pathology and Dermatology, Universidad Peruana Cayetano Heredia, Lima, Peru
Houston, USA

© Springer Science+Business Media New York 2015
V. G. Prieto (ed.), *Precision Molecular Pathology of Dermatologic Diseases,*
Molecular Pathology Library 9, DOI 10.1007/978-1-4939-2861-3_5

and specific—even allowing species identification—and do not require microbial growth in cultures [2]. They can be applied to formalin-fixed paraffin-embedded (FFPE) tissue [3]. Although these methodologies nowadays require substantial equipment and technical sophistication, making them expensive, it is expected that they will become cheaper and widely available in the future. This will be especially useful in this era of new and reemergent infectious diseases [4].

Molecular Tests Commonly Used in the Dermatopathology Practice

Signal Amplification Methods: In situ Hybridization

In situ hybridization (ISH) is a signal amplification-based test routinely used in the dermatopathology practice. The probes utilized are complementary RNA or DNA fragments labeled with chromogenic, fluorescent, or chemiluminescent tags. This method does not require the amplification of the target nucleic acid and therefore the chance of contamination with amplicons (i.e., PCR products) is low. ISH has the big advantage of allowing the concurrent examination of the tissue of interest.

Target Amplification Methods: Polymerase Chain Reaction

Polymerase chain reaction (PCR) is the most popular target amplification method. It is extremely sensitive, allowing the identification of very small numbers of microorganisms. Due to this high sensitivity, false positive results may be seen when contaminant DNA or dead microorganisms are present in the sample or in the laboratory environment. The PCR-based methods require expensive laboratory settings and therefore are not universally available in clinical dermatopathology laboratories.

Many variants of these methodologies may be applied to the investigation of infectious microorganisms. Real-time quantitative PCR (qPCR) is used to determine microbial load. Multiplex PCR allows the rapid detection of multiple microorganisms [5]. Nested PCR reduces interference and may indicate viability of the identified microorganisms [6]. Other modifications of PCR-based methods have been designed to provide rapid tests for clinical use [7, 8].

Viral Infections

Human Papillomavirus

The human papillomavirus (HPV) group comprises more than 100 serotypes [9]. HPV from the genera *alpha*, *beta*, *gamma*, *mu*, and *nu* can infect keratinocytes and cause a variety of cutaneous lesions in humans, including warts, condylomata, epidermodysplasia verruciformis, dysplasia, and squamous cell carcinoma (SCC) among others [10]. Immunosuppressed (e.g. organ transplant recipients) patients are at a higher risk of infection [11, 12].

ISH studies may become helpful when HPV is suspected in a skin biopsy [13]. Two sets of probes against low-risk (serotypes 6, 11, 42, 43, and 44) and high-risk (serotypes 16, 18, 31, 33, 35, 39, 45, 51, 52, 56, and 66) are routinely used at our institution. Examination of positive and negative controls along with correlation with histology is necessary to correctly interpret the test.

Several PCR-based tests have been developed to detect HPV. The sensitivity of these methods varies between 1 and 100,000 HPV genome copies per reaction [14]. Most of these studies are applicable to FFPE tissue [15]. These methods utilize standard or nested PCR [16, 17] and different amplicon genotyping systems such as direct sequencing [18, 19] (Fig. 5.1), restriction enzyme cleavage (RFLP) [20], reverse line blot [16], bead-based multiplex [21], and DNA microarray (APEX) [22] among others. Recently, novel methodologies for the detection of multiple cutaneous HPV using either different set of PCR primers [23] or multiplex genotyping (Luminex) [14, 24] have been reported (Fig. 5.1). Microarray-based HPV tests, some commercially available, have shown comparable results to PCR-based methods [9].

The interpretation of a molecular-based positive test in a skin biopsy requires correlation with the histological appearance of the lesion. Of note, although the risk of development of cutaneous SCC is higher in the immunosuppressed population [25] and HPV DNA has been detected in primary and metastatic SCC [26], both facts indicating a possible pathogenic link between HPV and nonmelanoma skin cancers, the role of HPV in cutaneous SCC induction remains unclear [27].

Human Herpesvirus

Herpes Simplex/Varicella Zoster

Molecular techniques can be helpful in the diagnosis of atypical herpes virus infections. Conventional microscopic findings in these cases may not be specific and immunohistochemical studies depend on the presence of infected cells in the sections examined.

ISH techniques have been used for the identification of varicella zoster virus in FFPE tissue [28]. Routine PCR-based methods performed on biopsies [29] and swab samples are being increasingly used to detect herpes virus DNA [30]. A proposed algorithm is to use immunofluorescent tests—which are cheaper and faster—at first screening and then run PCR on negative samples [31]. The use of internal controls is emphasized in order to rule out false negative results [32].

Multiplex reverse transcriptase PCR (RT-PCR) has been applied to detect herpesvirus-derived transcripts, [33] even in dried crusts or scales [34]. This method has the advantage of detecting nuclear RNAs or mRNAs, ensuring the pathogenic role of the virus in the disease [34].

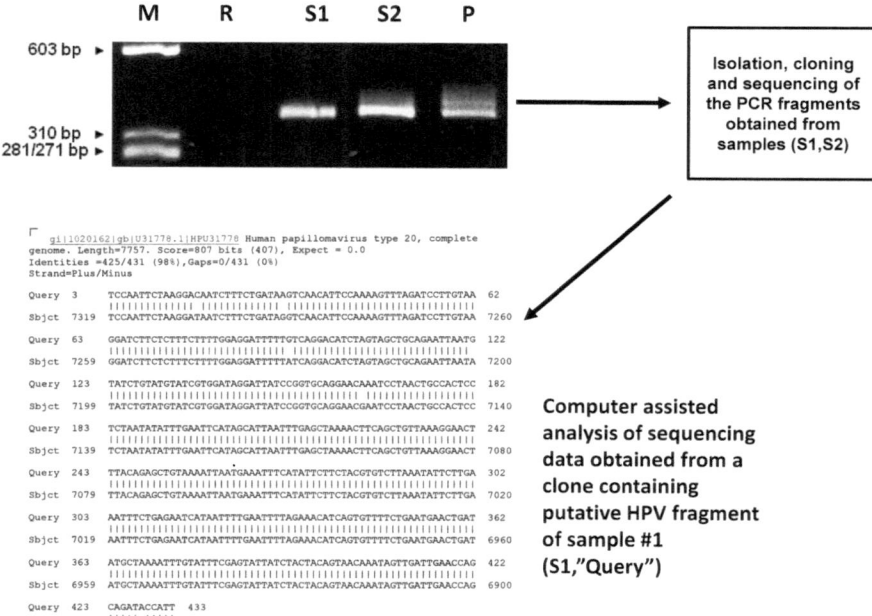

Fig. 5.1 Example of HPV testing using computer assisted analysis of HPV-PCR fragments obtained from skin lesions. Lanes: *M* DNA molecular weight marker (φx174 RF DNA), *R* reagent control, *S1* and *S2* samples from the patient, *P* HPV positive control DNA HPV-PCR fragments generated by nested EV-HPV PCR assay system [17] can be seen in the specimens (*S1* and *S2*) and in the positive DNA control. The HPV fragments from the specimens were cloned into a PCR cloning vector. Several HPV fragment containing clones were isolated and the purified plasmids were sent for sequencing. The clones from samples (*S1* and *S2*) showed high homology (98 %) to the HPV 20 prototype DNA sequences (NCBI-GenBank). In accordance with established guidelines, a nucleotide sequence was identified as an HPV type if it shared over 90 % L1 region homology with a known type of HPV from the databank. Interpretation of the HPV testing result: Infection with HPV type 20 was detected in the skin lesions. (Courtesy of Dr. Stephen K. Tyring and Dr. Peter Rady, Center for Clinical Studies, Houston, TX)

Epstein–Barr Virus

Epstein–Barr virus (EBV, human herpesvirus 4) cutaneous infection is associated with multiple disorders, ranging from acute syndromes such as infectious mononucleosis, Gianotti–Crosti syndrome, and Kikuchi disease to chronic infections such as hydroa vacciniforme, hypersensitivity to mosquito bites, and oral hairy leukoplakia [35]. B-, T-, and NK-lymphoproliferative disorders and lymphomas are also associated with EBV infection.

Immunohistochemical studies for detection of EBV viral proteins (EBNA1, EBNA2, LMP1, LMP2, among others) are used in some instances. The interpretation of these stains should always be made in the context of the histological findings, since in some EBV-related conditions the expression of these proteins may be only focal or even undetectable by immunohistochemistry.

Fig. 5.2 Cutaneous extra-nodal NK/T cell lymphoma, nasal type. This skin biopsy shows positive cells for EBER, as occurs in most of these aggressive lymphomas (EBER in situ hybridization (ISH), 10x)

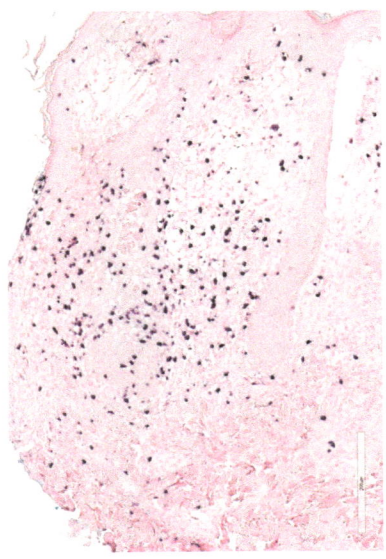

EBV-encoded RNAs (*EBER1* and *EBER2*) are transcripts associated with latent infection that are expressed in very high levels in virtually all infected cells [36]. *EBER* ISH is regarded as the gold standard assay for defining a lesion as EBV-related [36] (Fig. 5.2). False positive interpretations have been related to nonspecific staining and cross-reactivity with other materials [37]. False negative results due to RNA degradation can be avoided by running a parallel internal control [38]. It is important to consider that rare conditions, such as oral hairy leukoplakia shows downregulation of *EBER*; [39] again, interpretation of the test should be done correlating the results with the histopathological findings.

PCR amplification of latent EBV transcripts using RNA extracted from crusts of hydroa vacciniforme patients has been reported [40]. qPCR can be applied to identify EBV DNA; [41] the quantification of EBV DNA using qPCR on biopsies has been used for determination of viral load [42]. Detection of EBV DNA by PCR methods can be advantageous over *EBER* ISH in cases in which there is poor quality RNA or the EBV infection lacks *EBER* transcripts [36].

EBV episomal DNA, which is passed from infected cells to their daughters, is used as a marker for tumor clonality. Southern blot assays of the viral terminal repeat fragment (unique for every infecting EBV virion) will show a single band in cases of malignant neoplasms, thus demonstrating a monoclonal proliferation [43].

Human Herpesvirus 8

Immunohistochemical studies using monoclonal antibodies directed against human herpesvirus 8 (HHV-8) latent nuclear antigen-1 have been demonstrated to be 99% sensitive and 100% specific for Kaposi sarcoma lesions [44, 45].

PCR assays are both highly sensitive and specific for the detection of HHV-8 and permit quantitation of viral load [46, 47]. One caveat in the interpretation of these molecular tests is the detection of HHV-8 DNA in skin lesions due to concurrent viremia and not due to viral replication within lesional cells [48]. Correlation with histological and immunohistochemical findings is needed for an adequate interpretation of molecular tests results.

Human Polyomavirus

The demonstration of Merkel cell polyomavirus (MCV) DNA integration into about 80 % of Merkel cell carcinomas (MCC) [49] started a new exciting era for the virus-induced cancer pathogenesis field. It seems that MCC tumors may have different behavior depending on the presence or absence of MCV [50].

To date, nine human polyomaviruses are known. Besides MCV (the fifth identified polyomavirus), four other polyomaviruses have been identified: HPyV6 and HPyV7 as part of common skin flora, [51] TSaPyV in lesions of virus-associated trichodysplasia spinulosa, [52] and HPyV9 in serum of a kidney transplant patient [53].

Immunohistochemical methods can detect MCV proteins in most MCCs [54]. These methods use antibodies directed against MCV large T antigen (LT) [55]. Some cases, positive for MCV by PCR, may be negative for LT expression by immunohistochemistry [56]. A subset of these cases expresses MCV small T antigen (sT) [57].

MCV DNA detection by PCR is a very sensitive method. However, viral DNA can be detected from nontumoral tissue [58] since MCV may be found as normal flora of the skin [59].

Human T cell Lymphotropic Virus Type 1

Skin infection by human T cell lymphotropic virus type 1 (HTLV-1) is associated with infective dermatitis and adult T cell leukemia/lymphoma (ATLL) [60]. It is possible that HTLV-1-infected cells, along with activated T cells, infiltrate the skin of patients with infective dermatitis [61, 62]. This disease is considered as an early marker for the development of ATLL [63, 64].

The identification of integrated HTLV-1 proviral sequences in ATLL tumor cells has been extensively documented [65]. Cutaneous tumors in ATLL may be clinically and histopathologically indistinguishable from HTLV-1-negative lymphomas [66]. Besides serology, demonstration of monoclonal HTLV-1 proviral integration by Southern blot can be helpful in the diagnosis of ATLL [67]. Other cutaneous T cell lymphomas have been shown to lack HTLV-1 proviral DNA integration [68]. HTLV-1 proviral DNA load seem to be higher in smoldering ATLL than cutaneous ATLL, the last possibly representing a separate clinical entity [69]. RT-PCR can be used to identify the HTLV-1 *tax* and basic leucine zipper factor *(HBZ)* transcripts [70].

ISH using a HTLV-1 proviral probe has been applied to FFPE tissue sections to identify HTLV-1 proviral DNA, with reported better results than PCR [71]. More recently, ISH using a peptide nucleic acid (PNA) probe directed against the HTLV-1 *HBZ* gene (whose transcripts have been detected in all ATLL cells [72]) has been found to be a reliable test for HTLV-1 detection in pathology samples [70].

Bacterial Infections

Mycobacteria

Mycobacterium tuberculosis

Tuberculosis continues to be a health problem around the world, affecting not only developing countries but also showing increasing incidence in countries like England [73]. Diagnosis is always based on the isolation of *Mycobacterium tuberculosis* on culture, not a difficult task if the material is sputum, but quite difficult in the case of tegument tissues such as pleura or skin. Even the visualization of the bacteria on regular tissue cuts becomes problematic in such organs; therefore it is clear that better diagnostic methods are required in particular cases.

Nucleic acid amplification tests (NAATs) are designed to detect the smallest amount of either DNA or RNA through the amplification of specific sequences to the point of allowing detection by blotting [73]. PCR-based methods are now commercially available for the diagnosis of tuberculosis. These include the Roche Amplicor Mycobacterium tuberculosis test (PCR target amplification of part of the 16S rRNA gene, followed by the colorimetric detection of the PCR product) and the Gen-Probe Amplified Mycobacterium tuberculosis Direct Test (MTD), which is an isothermal transcription amplification method using ribosomal RNA (rRNA) as the target. A third method, called BD Probe Tec (multiple strand displacement system) uses isothermal amplification with DNA as substrate. Many institutions have also developed their own tests based on the IS6110 insertion sequence. Unfortunately, use of these tests also carries potential lack of specificity (since the same sequence is also present in other *Mycobacterium*) and sensitivity (since not all *M. tuberculosis* subtypes carry this sequence.) Other sequences used as target include MBP64, rpob and hsp65. Many of the methods now available also provide information regarding the sensitivity to drugs, such as rifampin, which is used as a criterion for the diagnosis of multidrug-resistant tuberculosis (MDRTB).

Most NAATs have used sputum samples and none of them is currently approved for its use in fixed tissue. Even more, lack of standardization of PCR methods performed of FFPE tissue makes interpretation of the results quite difficult and may explain the variability in sensitivity and specificity when these methods are applied to the diagnosis of tuberculosis in extrapulmonary sites such as lymph nodes [74,

75], pleura [76, 77], and skin [78–80]. Noteworthy is the fact that PCR may lack sensitivity under these circumstances, a concept not usually associated with the method. Possible explanations may include the presence of tissue inhibitors and lost of viability of the genetic material in old formalin-fixed tissue [81].

All said, the study of entities, such as tuberculides, by using PCR-based methods has been crucial for a better understanding of the physiopathology of tuberculosis affecting non-pulmonary organs. The study by Baselga [82] on PCR in the diagnosis of erythema induratum of Bazin helped to develop the concept of cutaneous tuberculosis as a spectrum whose ends are the multibacillary and paucibacillary forms, with distinct clinical presentations. Molecular biology applied to the study of tuberculosis helps us not only as a diagnostic test but also as a tool to reformulate our concepts of the disease.

Mycobacterium leprae

Molecular studies are especially helpful in the diagnosis of *Mycobacterium leprae* infections, since the bacteria cannot be cultured in artificial media. Clinical presentation and demonstration of acid-fast bacilli in smear preparations or skin biopsies are routinely used for diagnosis. Traditional methods, however, require at least 10^4 organisms/g of tissue to obtain reliable results [83]. In paucibacillary presentations of the disease (tuberculoid, some indeterminate forms) therefore, the bacilli are particularly difficult to demonstrate. PCR-based methods have long been used for detection of *M. leprae* [84, 85].

A nested PCR assay developed and tested at the Centers for Disease Control utilizing four nested primers, designed to amplify portions of the *M. leprae* groEL gene (corresponding to sequences found in *M. leprae* gene but not in *M. tuberculosis*) produced a result within 8 h. Positive signals for *M. leprae* could be achieved with just 0.003 pg of genomic DNA and as few as 20 organisms in crude lysates. The use of nested primers reduces nonspecific amplification, with increased sensitivity due to replenishment of reagents after every 25 cycles, and increased specificity as four primers need to bind for there to be successful amplification [84]. An RT-PCR detection system targeting the 16S rRNA of M. leprae improves on this sensitivity, making it possible to detect as few as 10 organisms in crude lysates. In this system, 53 % of specimens negative by smear are positive by RT-PCR. Furthermore, due to the rapid degradation of 16S rRNA on mycobacterial cell death, an rRNA-based detection system can distinguish between viable and nonviable *M. leprae*, and can thus be helpful in assessing the efficacy of instituted medications [86]. This is a key concern in leprosy where active mycobacterial infection versus persistent skin changes in the absence of infection with improved immunity can be challenging to discern (type 1 reaction). Furthermore, nested PCR protocols have been utilized in the differentiation between *M. leprae* and the newly described *Mycobacterium lepromatosis*, of clinical importance due to the tendency for the angioinvasive *M. lepromatosis* to cause a type of diffuse lepromatous leprosy with severe vascular involvement, namely Lucio phenomenon, which is usually associated with higher mortality [87, 88].

Staphylococcus aureus

Staphylococcus aureus is a pathogenic bacteria, with a wide variety of presentations in the skin, including superficial infections such as impetigo and folliculitis and deep infection including ecthyma, cellulitis, and abscess formation [89]. *S. aureus* is an angioinvasive bacteria which causes secondary skin involvement in bacteremia and is frequently implicated in chronic inflammatory conditions, such as dissecting cellulitis of the scalp and hidradenitis suppurativa, contributing to the morbidity of the disease. Targeting bacterial resistance mechanisms and testing drug susceptibility is key to the management of *S. aureus* infections. Methicillin-resistant S. aureus (MRSA) was first described in 1961, and its prevalence in both community and healthcare settings continues to increase [90]. The *mecA* gene encodes PBP-2a, a penicillin-binding protein that confers resistance to methicillin and related beta lactam antibiotics [91, 92]. The *mecA* gene belongs to a chromosomal element, the staphylococcal cassette chromosome (SCC*mec*). The protein A (SpA) virulence factor is encoded by the *spa* gene, enabling *S. aureus* to evade host immune responses. There is high variability of gene sequences within the Xr region of the *spa* gene, which is thus used to type strains [93]. Multiple qPCR kits are commercially available for the detection of MRSA, such as the MRSA diagnostic assay for Skin and Soft Tissue Infection (Xpert™, Cepheid, Sunnyvale, California) [94]. In bone and joint infection samples tested with Xpert™, the sensitivity and specificity for the detection of MRSA were both 100 %, with Gram stains positive in only 33 % of cases, and a median turn around time of 72 min compared to 79 h for culture [95]. The Xpert™ kit is a multiplex PCR assay that simultaneously detects three targets (*spa*, SCC*mec*, and *mecA*) within MRSA. It is able to distinguish between staphylococcal infections (MRSA, methicillin sensitive *S. aureus*, coagulase negative staphylococci) with its main limitation being its primer sets limited to staphylococcal organisms and thus inapplicability to a wider range of bacterial infections.

Treponema pallidum

The rate of primary and secondary syphilis in 2013 was double the lowest ever rate in 2001, representing a reemergence of this disease [96]. The causative agent, *Treponema pallidum* cannot be cultured in vitro. Darkfield microscopy for direct visualization of spirochetes and serologic antibody tests during early phases of disease, have low sensitivity and specificity [97]. Immunofluorescence staining methods have long been used in the detection of *T. pallidum*. A fluorescent antibody test applied to tissue fixed in formalin has significantly improved the detection of *T. pallidum*, but its limitation is that it requires experienced analysts for interpretation [98, 99]. Immunohistochemical assays utilizing monoclonal or polyclonal antibodies are sensitive, but can produce false positives in the setting of other spirochetes including Borrelia species with increased specificity when anti-*T. pallidum* antibodes are used [100, 101]. Molecular methods that amplify PCR products have been examined, but are limited by poor specificity [102]. In one such study the sensitivity for PCR detection of *T.*

pallidum was 75% compared to 91% with immunohistochemistry [101, 103]. This study used primers to amplify a 260 based pair (bp) fragment of the gene encoding the integral membrane lipoprotein of *T. pallidum*, with PCR products hybridized to the *tp47* gene (which does not have homology to any bacterial or eucaryotal proteins) between the 658 and 648 bp by Southern blot. PCR and immunohistochemistry were performed in the same sample in this study, indicating that combining the two methods may optimize sensitivity and specificity of *T. pallidum* detection.

Fungal Infections

Superficial Fungal Infections

Dermatophytoses are common superficial fungal infections limited to the keratinized integument, that is, the nail, stratum corneum of skin and hair. They are caused primarily by fungi of the genera *Trichophyton, Epidermophyton,* and *Microsporum.* Regardless of the causative species, dermatophytoses are characteristically either pruritic or scaly eruptions, although more protean and widespread presentations may be seen in the immunocompromised host. Whereas dermatophytes have low pathogenicity, persistent infection has adverse effects on the quality of life [104]. Furthermore, dermatophyte infection frequently results in a compromised skin barrier creating a portal of entry for other pathogens, with tinea pedis strongly associated with bacterial cellulitis of the lower limb [105]. It can be particularly difficult to identify the causative microorganism in nail fungal infections which are exquisitely recalcitrant to topical therapy. Traditional methods for detection include light microscopic analysis of wet preparations of involved tissue, such as nail clippings, incubated with potassium hydroxide to digest keratin, leaving the fungal chitinous wall intact. Artifacts are difficult to distinguish from fungal elements complicating interpretation, with a sensitivity between 83 and 88% and specificity of 84–95% in some studies [106, 107]. Another popular method is to expose nail clippings treated with KOH, or biopsy specimens stained with the PAS to the calcofluor white or blankophor fluorescent stains which bind to the fungal wall polysaccharide chitin, made of glucosamine residues, and enhance the contrast between fungal walls and artifactual debris. The reported sensitivity and specificity with calcofluor white with these methods ranges from 80 to 92% and 72 to 95% respectively [106–109]. A pitfall is that protozoa are also highlighted by calcofluor white, although morphology is helpful in distinguishing the two entities [110]. Culture remains the gold standard for fungal speciation. The problem with culture as a gold standard is the possibility of fungal contaminants during culture, fastidious and slow growing fungi resulting in false negatives (as high as 30%), and delayed results following laborious culture protocols [111]. The correct identification of the causative microorganism in onychomycosis, for example, is of importance, as *Trichophyton rubrum* is susceptible to oral terbinafine, whereas *Candida* spp. are not. Fluconazole is efficacious for candidal onychomycosis and itraconazole is recommended for onychomycosis due to nondermatophyte molds such as *Scytalidium* spp. [112].

Trichophyton rubrum

T. rubrum is most frequently implicated in superficial fungal infections [113]. Timely and targeted therapy would be aided by rapid and accurate diagnostic techniques. A two step, 15-min procedure for extraction of DNA from nail specimens followed by multiplex PCR has been designed [5, 114]. This duplex protocol uses two primers: one detecting the conserved DNA fragment encoding chitin synthetase 1 against dermatophytes in general, designed based on nucleotide sequencing of different dermatophytes found in the NCBI nucleotide database, and the second against the internal transcribed spacer 2 (a species specific ribosomal transcript region) for *T. rubrum*, and tested on dermatophyte and nondermatophyte reference strains and clinical isolates [115, 116]. Thus, a dermatophyte will show a positive band at the pandermatophyte 366 bp, and if that dermatophyte is *T. rubrum*, there will also be a strong positive band at the 203 bp. This PCR protocol has been externally validated, with 44 % of samples positive for dermatophyte by PCR compared to 34 % by culture. PCR also confirmed *T. rubrum* in 98 % of previously cultured cases. The kit is commercially available with positive and internal controls provided by the manufacturer (Dermatophyte PCR kit, Statens Serum Institut, Copenhagen, Denmark) requiring 1 day for laboratory diagnosis [117].

Deep Fungal Infections

Deep fungal infections can be categorized as primary pathogens that are inherently virulent, and secondary or opportunistic pathogens that are pathogenic in the context of an immunocompromised host. Timely diagnosis is crucial and targeted therapy based on species identification may be life saving. Concomitant culture and culture independent assays, such as galactomannan and $(1\rightarrow3)$-β-D-glucan antigen testing, of blood (unfortunately frequently negative in invasive fungal infection) and other accessible compartments in conjunction with biopsy of involved skin are key, with the goal being rapid detection and source control. For evaluation of cutaneous infection, whether primary or secondary, the conventional diagnostic approaches are tissue culture and histopathological examination. The same limitations identified in superficial fungal infections regarding sensitivity, specificity, interobserver variability, and lead time to diagnosis apply when evaluating deep fungal infections [118]. Successful identification on histopathology alone often depends on the abundance of organisms and the stage of infection. Additionally, a fungal organism may be visible on histopathology, but its identification may be limited if fresh tissue was not submitted for culture simultaneously. In cases where there was no isolation of organism on culture or there are significant discrepancies between the organism growing in culture and that seen on histopathology, doubts may rise about the certainty of the actual pathogen. Molecular techniques that can be evaluated in conjunction with skin biopsies are thus attractive.

Aspergillus spp

Analysis from 23 transplant centers in the USA revealed invasive aspergillosis to be the most commonly encountered invasive fungal infection in the hematopoetic stem cell transplant population, surpassing invasive candidiasis [119]. Of note, non-fumigatus *Aspergillus* species resistant to conventional amphotericin, such as *Aspergillus terreus*, are becoming increasingly prevalent [120]. A plethora of publications exist evaluating molecular methods for rapid detection of *Aspergillus* spp. Nucleic acid amplification based methods including nested PCR, qPCR, multiplex PCR followed by DNA microarray, and sequencing based methods in theory allow detection, identification, and strain typing [118].

These methods are designed as broad spectrum fungal detection systems, using conserved sequences to identify a broad range of fungal species, yet enough polymorphisms to simultaneously allow species identification [121]. The source material can be fresh tissue or paraffin embedded tissue but processing unavoidably destroys architecture and morphology (e.g., pattern of septation and branching of filamentous fungi). In practice, these methods often rely on mechanical methods to disrupt the fungal cell wall to access DNA for extraction that pose a risk of carry over contamination and the potential for contaminated reagents, and are not standardized for clinical sample size required for sensitivity of detection, test performance (sensitivity, specificity), and interpretation of results [122]. Combinations of analyte specific reagents (Luminex Molecular Diagnostics, Toronto, Canada) can be customized to test for a panel of regionally relevant fungi and can be tailored for testing of solid and liquid media. For example, an 11 plex panel representing 11 common clinically relevant molds, 4 of which were *Aspergillus* spp., has been tested using the Luminex multiplex PCR incubated with primer pairs for the 11 molds, followed by hybridization to microbead bound capture probes for fluorescence-based detection from fresh tissue samples [123]. Coinfection with multiple fungi can be detected by this method, if they are represented in the primer sets.

Fungal identification by comparison of the test fungus's characteristic protein expression pattern with species specific pattern expression through matrix assisted laser desorption/ionization time of flight mass spectrometry(MALDI-TOF-MS) is commercially available (Bruker Maldi Biotyper CA System, Bruker Daltonik, Germany) [124, 125]. This technique relies on standardized protein extraction practices to generate reproducible profiles [126]. This technique fails to adequately address mixed fungal infections, but can be used to assess drug sensitivity, by comparing changes in the spectra on exposure to the drug [127]. Fluorescence in situ hybridization (FISH) methodologies to localize fungal rRNA to pathology on FFPE tissue are being explored and are highly attractive for their ability to examine pathogens in histopathologic context with preservation of tissue architecture and pathogen morphology. However, current data suggest that PCR techniques are more sensitive than FISH in detecting invasive fungi. Current FISH methodologies broadly target fungal rRNA, the most conserved nucleic acid sequences, with modifications, such as utilization of locked nucleic acids which hybridize strongly to their complements and are thermally stable [128]. Weak signaling when rRNA is not abundant or probes are inadequately developed are potential pitfalls. Poor performance of ISH methods in necrotic tissue is also a limitation, however, FISH remains a promising option [129].

Alternaria spp

Alternaria is a ubiquitous pigmented fungus, found as spores in soil, air, and plants that typically do not cause infection in humans, with infection often occurring in the setting of traumatic inoculation [130]. It is an emerging fungal pathogen, rapidly fatal in immunosuppressed hosts although itraconazole may be effective when rapidly initiated. A rapid growing mold which may or may not be pigmented is identified on culture; however, failure to sporulate or pigment on multiple media is a frequently encountered problem, making culture-based identification almost impossible [131]. Furthermore, the most clinically relevant species, *Alternaria alternata* and *Alternaria infectoria* are not pigmented in tissue, thus a phaeohyphomycosis is unlikely to be considered even if the large yeast or septate hyphae are identified on histopathological examination. Successful identification of *Alternaria* spp. by amplification and subsequent sequencing of the Internal transcribed spacer (ITS) of the rRNA after failure to identify the mold evident on culture or on special stain analysis with PAS and GMS has been reported in multiple cases and illustrates the pivotal diagnostic role molecular methods can play [130–134].

Parasitic Diseases

Leishmaniasis

A great example of the utility of molecular techniques in diagnosing infectious diseases applies to leishmaniasis, the third most common vector transmitted disease worldwide. When dealing with tegumentary leishmaniasis, one has to confront a variety of clinical presentations, some of them easily confused with various other processes, infectious or not. To construct a solid diagnosis of tegumentary leishmaniasis it is required to visualize the parasite, either by direct exam of a smear, isolation in culture or by conventional histology in biopsy material. Indirect techniques, such as the intradermal test or Montenegro reaction, are significant when dealing with patients that are foreign to the endemic areas, but not in natives. The interpretation of smear preparations requires expertise, something expected in laboratory workers of endemic areas but unlikely in other locations. This last situation is far from being

Fig. 5.3 Gel electrophoresis showing PCR amplification of kinetoplastid DNA (kDNA) specific for *Leishmania* spp. Lane 1 shows molecular weight control, lanes 2 and 3 are the patient samples, lanes 4 and 5 are positive and negative controls (Courtesy of Dr. J. Arevalo, Universidad Peruana Cayetano Heredia, Lima, Peru)

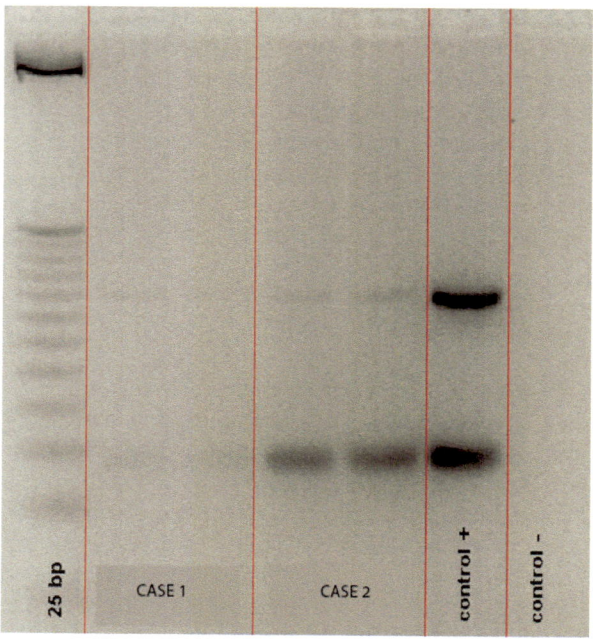

exceptional due to the increasing number of cutaneous leishmaniasis seen in travelers, such as tourists or army personnel, thus the increasing importance of molecular methods for diagnosis.

The molecular technique most commonly used is PCR amplification of specific primers targeting either the kinetoplast or rRNA gene (Fig. 5.3), ITS, mini-exon genes, and specific gene sequences (e.g., glycoproteins, heat shock proteins, and cysteine proteinases) [135]. Multiple publications have corroborated the validity of the method for diagnostic purposes [136, 137]. The technique has been simplified to make it more accessible to the caregivers in primary care settings [138–141]. qPCR can provide additional information, such as parasitic load or determination of species, contributing to the treatment strategies as well as to epidemiology studies on this subject [142, 143]. As the response to medical treatment may vary depending on the species of *Leishmania* involved, the utility of molecular biology becomes more manifest when assisting such species identification [144, 145].

Onchocerciasis

Filariasis is caused by nematodes (round worms) which parasitize humans, residing in the lymphatics and subcutaneous tissue with resultant lymphedema and cutaneous lesions. Over 120 million people worldwide are affected by filariasis which can be extremely disfiguring and disabling [146]. Early institution of diethylcarbamazine during the microfilarial phase can effectively eradicate the nematode *Loa Loa*, whereas treatment with diethylcarbazine can cause life threatening systemic collapse when the infecting nematode is onchocerca, an adverse reaction known as the Mazotti reaction [147]. Thus, speciation of the causative nematode in filariasis is key for administration of the correct treatment. Traditional diagnosis of nematodes depends heavily on morphology, specifically, by recognition of microfilaria on skin biopsies and thick blood smears. These methods are labor intensive, time consuming, and require experienced microscopists who can discern between the multiple species present in a region and between coinfecting nematodes in the same individual, making accuracy challenging [148, 149]. Antibody testing has its pitfalls, for example, an enzyme linked immunosorbent assay (ELISA) was unsuccessful in Brazil due to cross reactivity between *Onchocerca volvulus* and *Mansonella ozzardi* [150]. A nested PCR protocol tested on skin biopsies and whole blood samples holds promise. In this protocol, four PCR primers with partial sequences for 18S (small subunit rRNA), ITS-1, 5.8S and ITS-2 are used, thus amplifying the ITS of filarial species [151, 152]. Differentiation between species and detection of coinfection is possible as the ITS regions vary between species and thus yields amplicons of different sizes on gel electrophoresis, for example, *O. volvulus* yields a 344 bp band [152]. Importantly, cross amplification does not occur with parasites of other species, and low level parasitemia can be detected with only 0.003 ng/μl of *Onchocerca* DNA needed for diagnosis, which corresponds to less than a microfilaria worm [153].

References

1. Pierard GE, Arrese JE, De Doncker P, Pierard-Franchimont C. Present and potential diagnostic techniques in onychomycosis. J Am Acad Dermatol. 1996;34(2 Pt 1):273–7.
2. Procop GW. Molecular diagnostics for the detection and characterization of microbial pathogens. Clin Infect Dis. 2007;45(Suppl 2):S99–S111.
3. Payne DA, Van der Straten M, Carrasco D, Tyring SK. Molecular diagnosis of skin-associated infectious agents. Arch Dermatol. 2001;137(11):1497–502.
4. Bravo F, Sanchez MR. New and re-emerging cutaneous infectious diseases in Latin America and other geographic areas. Dermatol Clin. 2003;21(4):655–68, viii.
5. Arabatzis M, Bruijnesteijn van Coppenraet LE, Kuijper EJ, et al. Diagnosis of common dermatophyte infections by a novel multiplex real-time polymerase chain reaction detection/identification scheme. Br J Dermatol. 2007;157(4):681–9.
6. Okeke CN, Tsuboi R, Kawai M, Hiruma M, Ogawa H. Isolation of an intron-containing partial sequence of the gene encoding dermatophyte actin (ACT) and detection of a fragment of the transcript by reverse transcription-nested PCR as a means of assessing the viability of dermatophytes in skin scales. J Clin Microbiol. 2001;39(1):101–6.
7. Beifuss B, Bezold G, Gottlober P, et al. Direct detection of five common dermatophyte species in clinical samples using a rapid and sensitive 24-h PCR-ELISA technique open to protocol transfer. Mycoses. 2011;54(2):137–45.
8. Bergmans AM, van der Ent M, Klaassen A, Bohm N, Andriesse GI, Wintermans RG. Evaluation of a single-tube real-time PCR for detection and identification of 11 dermatophyte species in clinical material. Clin Microbiol Infect. 2010;16(6):704–10.

9. Dalstein V, Merlin S, Bali C, Saunier M, Dachez R, Ronsin C. Analytical evaluation of the PapilloCheck test, a new commercial DNA chip for detection and genotyping of human papillomavirus. J Virol Methods. 2009;156(1–2):77–83.

10. Lebwohl MG, Rosen T, Stockfleth E The role of human papillomavirus in common skin conditions: current viewpoints and therapeutic options. Cutis. 2010;86(5):suppl 1–11. quiz suppl 12.

11. Ulrich C, Hackethal M, Meyer T, et al. Skin infections in organ transplant recipients. J Dtsch Dermatol Ges. 2008;6(2):98–105.

12. Diamantis ML, Richmond HM, Rady PL, et al. Detection of human papillomavirus in multiple eccrine poromas in a patient with chronic graft-vs-host disease and immunosuppression. Arch Dermatol. 2011;147(1):120–2.

13. Amortegui AJ, Meyer MP. In-situ hybridization for the diagnosis and typing of human papillomavirus. Clin Biochem. 1990;23(4):301–6.

14. Michael KM, Forslund O, Bacevskij O, et al. Bead-based multiplex genotyping of 58 cutaneous human papillomavirus types. J Clin Microbiol. 2011;49(10):3560–7.

15. Resnick RM, Cornelissen MT, Wright DK, et al. Detection and typing of human papillomavirus in archival cervical cancer specimens by DNA amplification with consensus primers. J Natl Cancer Inst. 1990;82(18):1477–84.

16. Brink AA, Lloveras B, Nindl I, et al. Development of a general-primer-PCR-reverse-line-blotting system for detection of beta and gamma cutaneous human papillomaviruses. J Clin Microbiol. 2005;43(11):5581–7.

17. Berkhout RJ, Tieben LM, Smits HL, Bavinck JN, Vermeer BJ, ter Schegget J. Nested PCR approach for detection and typing of epidermodysplasia verruciformis-associated human papillomavirus types in cutaneous cancers from renal transplant recipients. J Clin Microbiol. 1995;33(3):690–5.

18. Hagiwara K, Uezato H, Arakaki H, et al. A genotype distribution of human papillomaviruses detected by polymerase chain reaction and direct sequencing analysis in a large sample of common warts in Japan. J Med Virol. 2005;77(1):107–12.

19. Forslund O, Antonsson A, Nordin P, Stenquist B, Hansson BG. A broad range of human papillomavirus types detected with a general PCR method suitable for analysis of cutaneous tumours and normal skin. J Gen Virol. 1999;80(9):2437–43.

20. Rubben A, Kalka K, Spelten B, Grussendorf-Conen EI. Clinical features and age distribution of patients with HPV 2/27/57-induced common warts. Arch Dermatol Res. 1997;289(6):337–40.

21. Schmitt M, Bravo IG, Snijders PJ, Gissmann L, Pawlita M, Waterboer T. Bead-based multiplex genotyping of human papillomaviruses. J Clin Microbiol. 2006;44(2):504–12.

22. Gheit T, Billoud G, de Koning MN, et al. Development of a sensitive and specific multiplex PCR method combined with DNA microarray primer extension to detect Betapapillomavirus types. J Clin Microbiol. 2007;45(8):2537–44.

23. Sasagawa T, Mitsuishi T. Novel polymerase chain reaction method for detecting cutaneous human papillomavirus DNA. J Med Virol. 2012;84(1):138–44.

24. de Koning MN, ter Schegget J, Eekhof JA, et al. Evaluation of a novel broad-spectrum PCR-multiplex genotyping assay for identification of cutaneous wart-associated human papillomavirus types. J Clin Microbiol. 2010;48(5):1706–11.

25. Dubina M, Goldenberg G. Viral-associated nonmelanoma skin cancers: a review. Am J Dermatopathol. 2009;31(6):561–73.

26. Zaravinos A, Kanellou P, Spandidos DA. Viral DNA detection and RAS mutations in actinic keratosis and nonmelanoma skin cancers. Br J Dermatol. 2010;162(2):325–31.

27. zur Hausen H. Papillomaviruses in the causation of human cancers—a brief historical account. Virology. 2009;384(2):260–5.

28. Annunziato P, Lungu O, Gershon A, Silvers DN, LaRussa P, Silverstein SJ. In situ hybridization detection of varicella zoster virus in paraffin-embedded skin biopsy samples. Clin Diagn Virol. 1996;7(2):69–76.

29. Lilie HM, Wassilew SW, Wolff MH. Early diagnosis of herpes zoster by polymerase chain reaction. J Eur Acad Dermatol Venereol. 2002;16(1):53–7.

30. Boer A, Herder N, Blodorn-Schlicht N, Steinkraus V, Falk TM. Refining criteria for diagnosis of cutaneous infections caused by herpes viruses through correlation of morphology with molecular pathology. Indian J Dermatol Venereol Leprol. 2006;72(4):270–5.
31. Bezold G, Lange M, Gethoffer K, Gall H, Peter RU. Detection of cutaneous herpes simplex virus infections by immunofluorescence vs. PCR. J Eur Acad Dermatol Venereol. 2003;17(4):430–3.
32. Bezold G, Volkenandt M, Gottlober P, Peter RU. Detection of herpes simplex virus and varicella-zoster virus in clinical swabs: frequent inhibition of PCR as determined by internal controls. Mol Diagn. 2000;5(4):279–84.
33. Rahaus M, Desloges N, Wolff MH. Development of a multiplex RT-PCR to detect transcription of varicella-zoster virus encoded genes. J Virol Methods. 2003;107(2):257–60.
34. Yamamoto T, Yamada A, Tsuji K, Iwatsuki K. Tracing of the molecular remnants of herpes virus infections in necrotic skin tissue. Eur J Dermatol. 2008;18(5):499–503.
35. Mendoza N, Diamantis M, Arora A, et al. Mucocutaneous manifestations of Epstein-Barr virus infection. Am J Clin Dermatol. 2008;9(5):295–305.
36. Gulley ML, Tang W. Laboratory assays for Epstein-Barr virus-related disease. J Mol Diagn. 2008;10(4):279–92.
37. Gulley ML. Molecular diagnosis of Epstein-Barr virus-related diseases. J Mol Diagn. 2001;3(1):1–10.
38. Gulley ML, Glaser SL, Craig FE, et al. Guidelines for interpreting EBER in situ hybridization and LMP1 immunohistochemical tests for detecting Epstein-Barr virus in Hodgkin lymphoma. Am J Clin Pathol. 2002;117(2):259–67.
39. Gilligan K, Rajadurai P, Resnick L, Raab-Traub N. Epstein-Barr virus small nuclear RNAs are not expressed in permissively infected cells in AIDS-associated leukoplakia. Proc Natl Acad Sci U S A. 1990;87(22):8790–4.
40. Yamamoto T, Tsuji K, Suzuki D, Morizane S, Iwatsuki K. A novel, noninvasive diagnostic probe for hydroa vacciniforme and related disorders: detection of latency-associated Epstein-Barr virus transcripts in the crusts. J Microbiol Methods. 2007;68(2):403–407.
41. Kubota N, Wada K, Ito Y, et al. One-step multiplex real-time PCR assay to analyse the latency patterns of Epstein-Barr virus infection. J Virol Methods. 2008;147(1):26–36.
42. Ryan JL, Fan H, Glaser SL, Schichman SA, Raab-Traub N, Gulley ML. Epstein-Barr virus quantitation by real-time PCR targeting multiple gene segments: a novel approach to screen for the virus in paraffin-embedded tissue and plasma. J Mol Diagn. 2004;6(4):378–85.
43. Raab-Traub N, Flynn K. The structure of the termini of the Epstein-Barr virus as a marker of clonal cellular proliferation. Cell. 1986;47(6):883–9.
44. Robin YM, Guillou L, Michels JJ, Coindre JM. Human herpesvirus 8 immunostaining: a sensitive and specific method for diagnosing Kaposi sarcoma in paraffin-embedded sections. Am J Clin Pathol. 2004;121(3):330–4.
45. Patel RM, Goldblum JR, Hsi ED. Immunohistochemical detection of human herpes virus-8 latent nuclear antigen-1 is useful in the diagnosis of Kaposi sarcoma. Mod Pathol. 2004;17(4):456–60.
46. Nuovo M, Nuovo G. Utility of HHV8 RNA detection for differentiating Kaposi's sarcoma from its mimics. J Cutan Pathol. 2001;28(5):248–55.
47. Tedeschi R, Dillner J, De Paoli P. Laboratory diagnosis of human herpesvirus 8 infection in humans. Eur J Clin Microbiol Infect Dis. 2002;21(12):831–44.
48. Kazakov DV, Schmid M, Adams V, et al. HHV-8 DNA sequences in the peripheral blood and skin lesions of an HIV-negative patient with multiple eruptive dermatofibromas: implications for the detection of HHV-8 as a diagnostic marker for Kaposi's sarcoma. Dermatology. 2003;206(3):217–21.
49. Feng H, Shuda M, Chang Y, Moore PS. Clonal integration of a polyomavirus in human Merkel cell carcinoma. Science. 2008;319(5866):1096–100.
50. Duncavage EJ, Le BM, Wang D, Pfeifer JD. Merkel cell polyomavirus: a specific marker for Merkel cell carcinoma in histologically similar tumors. Am J Surg Pathol. 2009;33(12):1771–7.

51. Schowalter RM, Pastrana DV, Pumphrey KA, Moyer AL, Buck CB. Merkel cell polyomavirus and two previously unknown polyomaviruses are chronically shed from human skin. Cell Host Microbe. 2010;7(6):509–15.
52. van der Meijden E, Janssens RW, Lauber C, Bouwes Bavinck JN, Gorbalenya AE, Feltkamp MC. Discovery of a new human polyomavirus associated with trichodysplasia spinulosa in an immunocompromized patient. PLoS Pathog. 2010;6(7):e1001024.
53. Scuda N, Hofmann J, Calvignac-Spencer S, et al. A novel human polyomavirus closely related to the african green monkey-derived lymphotropic polyomavirus. J Virol. 2011;85(9):4586–90.
54. Busam KJ, Jungbluth AA, Rekthman N, et al. Merkel cell polyomavirus expression in merkel cell carcinomas and its absence in combined tumors and pulmonary neuroendocrine carcinomas. Am J Surg Pathol. 2009;33(9):1378–85.
55. Shuda M, Arora R, Kwun HJ, et al. Human Merkel cell polyomavirus infection I. MCV T antigen expression in Merkel cell carcinoma, lymphoid tissues and lymphoid tumors. Int J Cancer. 2009;125(6):1243–9.
56. Bhatia K, Goedert JJ, Modali R, Preiss L, Ayers LW. Immunological detection of viral large T antigen identifies a subset of Merkel cell carcinoma tumors with higher viral abundance and better clinical outcome. Int J Cancer. 2010;127(6):1493–6.
57. Shuda M, Kwun HJ, Feng H, Chang Y, Moore PS. Human Merkel cell polyomavirus small T antigen is an oncoprotein targeting the 4E-BP1 translation regulator. J Clin Invest. 2011;121(9):3623–34.
58. Loyo M, Guerrero-Preston R, Brait M, et al. Quantitative detection of Merkel cell virus in human tissues and possible mode of transmission. Int J Cancer. 2010;126(12):2991–6.
59. Foulongne V, Dereure O, Kluger N, Moles JP, Guillot B, Segondy M. Merkel cell polyomavirus DNA detection in lesional and nonlesional skin from patients with Merkel cell carcinoma or other skin diseases. Br J Dermatol. 2010;162(1):59–63.
60. Amano M, Setoyama M, Grant A, Kerdel FA. Human T-lymphotropic virus 1 (HTLV-1) infection–dermatological implications. Int J Dermatol. 2011;50(8):915–20.
61. Nobre V, Guedes AC, Martins ML, et al. Dermatological findings in 3 generations of a family with a high prevalence of human T cell lymphotropic virus type 1 infection in Brazil. Clin Infect Dis. 2006;43(10):1257–63.
62. Torres-Cabala CA, Curry JL, Li Ning Tapia EM, et al. HTLV-1-associated infective dermatitis demonstrates low frequency of FOXP3-positive T-regulatory lymphocytes. J Dermatol Sci. 2015;77(3):150–5.
63. Hanchard B, LaGrenade L, Carberry C, et al. Childhood infective dermatitis evolving into adult T-cell leukaemia after 17 years. Lancet. 1991;338(8782–8783):1593–94.
64. Lee R, Schwartz RA. Human T-lymphotrophic virus type 1-associated infective dermatitis: a comprehensive review. J Am Acad Dermatol. 2011;64(1):152–60.
65. Poiesz BJ, Ruscetti FW, Gazdar AF, Bunn PA, Minna JD, Gallo RC. Detection and isolation of type C retrovirus particles from fresh and cultured lymphocytes of a patient with cutaneous T-cell lymphoma. Proc Natl Acad Sci U S A. 1980;77(12):7415–9.
66. Shuh M, Beilke M. The human T-cell leukemia virus type 1 (HTLV-1): new insights into the clinical aspects and molecular pathogenesis of adult T-cell leukemia/lymphoma (ATLL) and tropical spastic paraparesis/HTLV-associated myelopathy (TSP/HAM). Microsc Res Tech. 2005;68(3–4):176–96.
67. Whittaker SJ, Ng YL, Rustin M, Levene G, McGibbon DH, Smith NP. HTLV-1-associated cutaneous disease: a clinicopathological and molecular study of patients from the U.K. Br J Dermatol. 1993;128(5):483–92.
68. Li G, Vowels BR, Benoit BM, Rook AH, Lessin SR. Failure to detect human T-lymphotropic virus type-I proviral DNA in cell lines and tissues from patients with cutaneous T-cell lymphoma. J Invest Dermatol. 1996;107(3):308–13.
69. Amano M, Kurokawa M, Ogata K, Itoh H, Kataoka H, Setoyama M. New entity, definition and diagnostic criteria of cutaneous adult T-cell leukemia/lymphoma: human T-lymphotropic virus type 1 proviral DNA load can distinguish between cutaneous and smoldering types. J Dermatol. 2008;35(5):270–5.

70. Shimizu-Kohno K, Satou Y, Arakawa F, et al. Detection of HTLV-1 by means of HBZ gene in situ hybridization in formalin-fixed and paraffin-embedded tissues. Cancer Sci. 2011;102(7):1432–6.
71. Arai E, Chow KC, Li CY, Tokunaga M, Katayama I. Differentiation between cutaneous form of adult T cell leukemia/lymphoma and cutaneous T cell lymphoma by in situ hybridization using a human T cell leukemia virus-1 DNA probe. Am J Pathol. 1994;144(1):15–20.
72. Satou Y, Yasunaga J, Yoshida M, Matsuoka M. HTLV-I basic leucine zipper factor gene mRNA supports proliferation of adult T cell leukemia cells. Proc Natl Acad Sci U S A. 2006;103(3):720–5.
73. Dinnes J, Deeks J, Kunst H, et al. A systematic review of rapid diagnostic tests for the detection of tuberculosis infection. Health Technol Assess. 2007;11(3):1–196.
74. Osores F, Nolasco O, Verdonck K, et al. Clinical evaluation of a 16S ribosomal RNA polymerase chain reaction test for the diagnosis of lymph node tuberculosis. Clin Infect Dis. 2006;43(7):855–9.
75. Cortez MV, Oliveira CM, Monte RL, et al. HIV-associated tuberculous lymphadenitis: the importance of polymerase chain reaction (PCR) as a complementary tool for the diagnosis of tuberculosis—a study of 104 patients. An Bras Dermatol. 2011;86(5):925–31.
76. Kumar P, Sen MK, Chauhan DS, Katoch VM, Singh S, Prasad HK. Assessment of the N-PCR assay in diagnosis of pleural tuberculosis: detection of *M. tuberculosis* in pleural fluid and sputum collected in tandem. PLoS ONE. 2010;5(4):e10220.
77. Hasaneen NA, Zaki ME, Shalaby HM, El-Morsi AS. Polymerase chain reaction of pleural biopsy is a rapid and sensitive method for the diagnosis of tuberculous pleural effusion. Chest. 2003;124(6):2105–11.
78. Abdalla CM, de Oliveira ZN, Sotto MN, Leite KR, Canavez FC, de Carvalho CM. Polymerase chain reaction compared to other laboratory findings and to clinical evaluation in the diagnosis of cutaneous tuberculosis and atypical mycobacteria skin infection. Int J Dermatol. 2009;48(1):27–35.
79. Hsiao PF, Tzen CY, Chen HC, Su HY. Polymerase chain reaction based detection of *Mycobacterium tuberculosis* in tissues showing granulomatous inflammation without demonstrable acid-fast bacilli. Int J Dermatol. 2003;42(4):281–6.
80. Padmavathy L, Rao L, Veliath A. Utility of polymerase chain reaction as a diagnostic tool in cutaneous tuberculosis. Indian J Dermatol Venereol Leprol. 2003;69(3):214–6.
81. Luo RF, Scahill MD, Banaei N. Comparison of single-copy and multicopy real-time PCR targets for detection of *Mycobacterium tuberculosis* in paraffin-embedded tissue. J Clin Microbiol. 2010;48(7):2569–70.
82. Baselga E, Margall N, Barnadas MA, Coll P, de Moragas JM. Detection of *Mycobacterium tuberculosis* DNA in lobular granulomatous panniculitis (erythema induratum-nodular vasculitis). Arch Dermatol. 1997;133(4):457–62.
83. Bang PD, Suzuki K, Phuong le T, Chu TM, Ishii N, Khang TH. Evaluation of polymerase chain reaction-based detection of *Mycobacterium leprae* for the diagnosis of leprosy. J Dermatol. 2009;36(5):269–76.
84. Plikaytis BB, Gelber RH, Shinnick TM. Rapid and sensitive detection of *Mycobacterium leprae* using a nested-primer gene amplification assay. J Clin Microbiol. 1990;28(9):1913–7.
85. de Wit MY, Douglas JT, McFadden J, Klatser PR. Polymerase chain reaction for detection of *Mycobacterium leprae* in nasal swab specimens. J Clin Microbiol. 1993;31(3):502–6.
86. Kurabachew M, Wondimu A, Ryon JJ. Reverse transcription-PCR detection of *Mycobacterium leprae* in clinical specimens. J Clin Microbiol. 1998;36(5):1352–6.
87. Han XY, Seo YH, Sizer KC, et al. A new Mycobacterium species causing diffuse lepromatous leprosy. Am J Clin Pathol. 2008;130(6):856–64.
88. Han XY, Sizer KC, Velarde-Felix JS, Frias-Castro LO, Vargas-Ocampo F. The leprosy agents Mycobacterium lepromatosis and Mycobacterium leprae in Mexico. Int J Dermatol. 2012;51(8):952–9.
89. Stevens DL, Bisno AL, Chambers HF, Dellinger EP, Goldstein EJ, Gorbach SL, Hirschmann JV, Kaplan SL, Montoya JG, Wade JC. Practice guidelines for the diagnosis and management of skin and soft tissue infections: 2014 update by the infectious diseases society of America. Clin Infect Dis. 2014;1–43.

90. Barber M. Methicillin-resistant staphylococci. J Clin Pathol. 1961;14(4):385-&.
91. Inglis B, Matthews PR, Stewart PR. The expression in Staphylococcus aureus of cloned DNA encoding methicillin resistance. J Gen Microbiol. 1988;134:1465–9.
92. Tesch W, Strassle A, Bergerbachi B, Ohara D, Reynolds P, Kayser FH. Cloning and expression of methicillin resistance from Staphylococcus epidermidis in Staphylococcus carnosus. Antimicrob Agents Chemother. 1988;32(10):1494–9.
93. Votintseva AA, Fung R, Miller RR, et al. Prevalence of Staphylococcus aureus protein A (spa) mutants in the community and hospitals in Oxfordshire. Bmc Microbiol. 2014;12:14.
94. Wolk DM, Picton E, Johnson D, et al. Multicenter evaluation of the Cepheid Xpert methicillin-resistant Staphylococcus aureus (MRSA) test as a rapid screening method for detection of MRSA in nares. J Clin Microbiol. 2009;47(3):758–64.
95. Dubouix-Bourandy A, de Ladoucette A, Pietri V, et al. Direct detection of Staphylococcus osteoarticular infections by use of Xpert MRSA/SA SSTI real-time PCR. J Clin Microbiol. 2011;49(12):4225–30.
96. Patton ME, Su JR, Nelson R, Weinstock H. Primary and secondary syphilis—United States, 2005–2013. Mmwr-Morb Mortal Wkly Rep. 2014;63(18):402–6.
97. Jethwa HS, Schmitz JL, Dallabetta G, et al. Comparison of molecular and microscopic techniques for detection of Treponema pallidum in genital ulcers. J Clin Microbiol. 1995;33(1):180–3.
98. Romanowski B, Forsey E, Prasad E, Lukehart S, Tam M, Hook EW. Detection of Treponema pallidum by a fluorescent monoclonal-antibody test. Sex Transm Dis. 1987;14(3):156–9.
99. Hunter EF, Greer PW, Swisher BL, et al. Immunofluorescent staining of treponema in tissues fixed with formalin. Arch Pathol Lab Med. 1984;108(11):878–80.
100. Hoang MP, High WA, Molberg KH. Secondary syphilis: a histologic and immunohisto-chemical evaluation. J Cutan Pathol. 2004;31(9):595–9.
101. Buffet M, Grange PA, Gerhardt P, et al. Diagnosing Treponema pallidum in secondary syphilis by PCR and immunohistochemistry. J Invest Dermatol. 2007;127(10):2345–50.
102. Kouznetsov AV, Weisenseel P, Trommler P, Multhaup S, Prinz JC. Detection of the 47-kilodalton membrane immunogen gene of Treponema pallidum in various tissue sources of patients with syphilis. Diagn Microbiol Infect Dis. 2005;51(2):143–5.
103. Deka RK, Machius M, Norgard MV, Tomchick DR. Crystal structure of the 47-kDa lipoprotein of Treponema pallidum reveals a novel penicillin-binding protein. J Biol Chem. 2002;277(44):41857–64.
104. Daniel RC. Onychomycosis: burden of disease and the role of topical antifungal treatment. J Drugs Dermatol. Nov 2013;12(11):1263–6.
105. Dalal AE-SM, Mimouni D, Ray S, Days W, Hodak E, Leibovici L, Paul M. Interventions for the prevention of recurrent erysipelas and cellulitis (Protocol). Cochrane Database of Systematic Reviews. 2012;(4):1–13.
106. Hamer EC, Moore CB, Denning DW. Comparison of two fluorescent whiteners, Calcofluor and Blankophor, for the detection of fungal elements in clinical specimens in the diagnostic laboratory. Clin Microb Infect. 2006;12(2):181–4.
107. Haldane DJM, Robart E. A comparison of calcofluor white, potassium hydroxide, and culture for the laboratory diagnosis of superficial fungal infection. Diagn Microbiol Infect Dis. 1990;13(4):337–9.
108. Mcnall EG, Sternberg TH, Newcomer VD, Sorensen LJ. Chemical and immunological studies on dermatophyte cell wall polysaccharides. J Invest Dermatol. 1961;36(2):155–7.
109. Weinberg JM, Koestenblatt EK, Tutrone WD, Tishler HR, Najarian L. Comparison of diagnostic methods in the evaluation of onychomycosis. J Am Acad Dermatol. 2003;49(2):193–7.
110. Luna VA, Stewart BK, Bergeron DL, Clausen CR, Plorde JJ, Fritsche TR. Use of the fluorochrome calcofluor white in the screening of stool specimens for spores of microsporidia. Am J Clin Pathol. 1995;103(5):656–9.
111. Gupta AK, Zaman M, Singh J. Diagnosis of Trichophyton rubrum from onychomycotic nail samples using polymerase chain reaction and calcofluor white microscopy. J Am Podiatr Med Assoc. 2008;98(3):224–8.
112. Elewski BE. Onychomycosis: pathogenesis, diagnosis, and management. Clin Microbiol Rev. 1998;11(3):415–29.

113. Havlickova B, Czaika VA, Friedrich M. Epidemiological trends in skin mycoses worldwide. Mycoses. 2008;51(Suppl 4):2–15. 2009;52(1):95.
114. Jensen RH, Arendrup MC. Molecular diagnosis of dermatophyte infections. Curr Opin Infect Dis. 2012;25(2):126–34.
115. Brillowska-Dabrowska A, Saunte DM, Arendrup MC. Five hour diagnosis of dermatophyte nail infections with specific detection of *Trichophton rubrum*. J Clin Microbiol. 2007;45(4):1200–4.
116. Kardjeva RS V, Kantardjiev T, Devliotou-Panagiotdou D, Sotiriou E, Graser Y. Forty-eight hour diagnosis of onychomycosis with subtyping of *Trichophyton rubrum* strains. J Clin Microbiol. 2006;44(4):1419–27.
117. Kondori N, Abrahamsson AL, Ataollahy N, Wenneras C. Comparison of a new commercial test, Dermatophyte-PCR kit, with conventional methods for rapid detection and identification of *Trichophyton rubrum* in nail specimens. Med Mycol. 2010;48(7):1005–8.
118. Baskova L, Buchta V. Laboratory diagnostics of invasive fungal infections: an overview with emphasis on molecular approach. Folia Microbiol. 2012;57(5):421–30.
119. Person AK, Kontoyiannis DP, Alexander BD. Fungal infections in transplant and oncology patients. Hematol Oncol Clin North Am. 2011;25(1):193-+.
120. Arendrup MC, Cuenca-Estrella M, Lass-Florl C, Hope WW, Suscep ECA. EUCAST technical note on aspergillus and amphotericin B, itraconazole, and posaconazole. Clin Microbiol Infec. 2012;18(7):E248–E250.
121. Olano JP, Walker DH. Diagnosing emerging and reemerging infectious diseases the pivotal role of the pathologist. Arch Pathol Lab Med. 2011;135(1):83–91.
122. Preuner S, Lion T. Towards molecular diagnostics of invasive fungal infections. Expert Rev Mol Diagn. 2009;9(5):397–401.
123. Babady NE, Miranda E, Gilhuley KA. Evaluation of luminex xTAG fungal analyte-specific reagents for rapid identification of clinically relevant fungi. J Clin Microbiol. 2011;49(11):3777–82.
124. Halliday CL, Kidd SE, Sorrell TC, Chen SC. Molecular diagnostic methods for invasive fungal disease: the horizon draws nearer. Pathology. 2015;3:257–69.
125. Schulthess B, Ledermann R, Mouttet F, et al. Use of the Bruker MALDI biotyper for identification of molds in the clinical mycology laboratory. J Clin Microbiol. 2014;52(8):2797–803.
126. Lau AF, Drake SK, Calhoun LB, Henderson CM, Zelazny AM. Development of a clinically comprehensive database and a simple procedure for identification of molds from solid media by matrix-assisted laser desorption ionization-time of flight mass spectrometry. J Clin Microbiol. 2013;51(3):828–34.
127. De Carolis EVA, Florio AR. Use of matrix-assisted laser desorption ionization-time of flight mass spectrometry for capsofungin susceptibility testing of candida and aspergillus species. J Clin Microbiol. 2012;2012(50):2479–83.
128. Kurreck J, Wyszko E, Gillen C, Erdmann VA. Design of antisense oligonucleotides stabilized by locked nucleic acids. Nucleic Acids Res. 2002;30(9):1911–8.
129. Montone KT, Guarner J. In situ hybridization for rRNA sequences in anatomic pathology specimens, applications for fungal pathogen detection: a review. Adv Anat Pathol. 2013;20(3):168–74.
130. Lo Cascio ML G, Maccacaro L, Fontana R. Utility of molecular identification in opportunistic mycotic infections: a case of cutaneous *Alternaria infectoria* infection in a cardiac transplant recipient. J Clin Microbiol. 2004;42(11):5334–6.
131. Daglar D, Akman-Karakas A, Ozhak-Baysan B, Gunseren F, Ciftcioglu MA, Buitrago MJ, Rodriguez-Tudela JL. Cutaneous *Alternaria infectoria* infection diagnosed by molecular techniques in a renal transplant patient. Clin Lab Publ. 2014;60:1569–72.
132. Williams C, Layton AM, Kerr K, Kibbler C, Barton RC. Cutaneous infection with an Alternaria sp. in an immunocompetent host. Clin Exp Dermatol. Jul 2008;33(4):440–2.
133. Gerdsen R, Uerlich M, De Hoog GS, Bieber T, Horre R. Sporotrichoid phaeohyphomycosis due to *Alternaria infectoria*. Br J Dermatol. 2001;145(3):484–6.
134. Robert T, Talarmin JP, Leterrier M, et al. Phaeohyphomycosis due to *Alternaria infectoria*: a single-center experience with utility of PCR for diagnosis and species identification. Med Mycol. 2012;50(6):594–600.

135. Reithinger R, Dujardin JC. Molecular diagnosis of leishmaniasis: current status and future applications. J Clin Microbiol. 2007;45(1):21–5.
136. Goto H, Lindoso JA. Current diagnosis and treatment of cutaneous and mucocutaneous leishmaniasis. Expert Rev Anti Infect Ther. 2010;8(4):419–33.
137. Andrade RV, Massone C, Lucena MN, et al. The use of polymerase chain reaction to confirm diagnosis in skin biopsies consistent with American tegumentary leishmaniasis at histopathology: a study of 90 cases. An Bras Dermatol. 2011;86(5):892–6.
138. Espinosa D, Boggild AK, Deborggraeve S, et al. Leishmania OligoC-TesT as a simple, rapid, and standardized tool for molecular diagnosis of cutaneous leishmaniasis in Peru. J Clin Microbiol. 2009;47(8):2560–3.
139. Deborggraeve S, Laurent T, Espinosa D, et al. A simplified and standardized polymerase chain reaction format for the diagnosis of leishmaniasis. J Infect Dis. 2008;198(10):1565–72.
140. Boggild AK, Valencia BM, Veland N, et al. Non-invasive cytology brush PCR diagnostic testing in mucosal leishmaniasis: superior performance to conventional biopsy with histopathology. PLoS ONE. 2011;6(10):e26395.
141. Boggild AK, Ramos AP, Valencia BM, et al. Diagnostic performance of filter paper lesion impression PCR for secondarily infected ulcers and nonulcerative lesions caused by cutaneous leishmaniasis. J Clin Microbiol. 2011;49(3):1097–100.
142. Kumar R, Bumb RA, Salotra P. Correlation of parasitic load with interleukin-4 response in patients with cutaneous leishmaniasis due to *Leishmania tropica*. FEMS Immunol Med Microbiol. 2009;57(3):239–46.
143. Schonian G, Kuhls K, Mauricio IL. Molecular approaches for a better understanding of the epidemiology and population genetics of Leishmania. Parasitology. 2011;138(4):405–25.
144. Arevalo J, Ramirez L, Adaui V, et al. Influence of Leishmania (Viannia) species on the response to antimonial treatment in patients with American tegumentary leishmaniasis. J Infect Dis. 2007;195(12):1846–51.
145. Alvarez P, Salinas C, Bravo F. Calcified bodies in New World cutaneous leishmaniasis. Am J Dermatopathol. 2011;33(8):827–30.
146. Global Programme to eliminate lymphatic filariasis. Progress report on mass drug administration, 2010. Wkly Epidemiol Rec. 2011;86(35):377–88.
147. Bryceson AD, Warrell DA, Pope HM. Dangerous reactions to treatment of onchocerciasis with diethylcarbamazine. Br Med J. 1977;1(6063):742–4.
148. Walther M, Muller R. Diagnosis of human filariases—(Except onchocerciasis). Adv Parasit. 2003;53:149–93.
149. Harnett W, Bradley JE, Garate T. Molecular and immunodiagnosis of human filarial nematode infections. Parasitology. 1998;117:S59–S71.
150. Shelley AJ, Coscaron S. Simuliid blackflies (Diptera: Simuliidae) and ceratopogonid midges (Diptera: Ceratopogonidae) as vectors of Mansonella ozzardi (Nematoda: Onchocercidae) in northern Argentina. Memorias do Instituto Oswaldo Cruz. 2001;96(4):451–8.
151. Morales-Hojas R, Post RJ, Shelley AJ, Maia-Herzog M, Coscaron S, Cheke RA. Characterisation of nuclear ribosomal DNA sequences from *Onchocerca volvulus* and *Mansonella ozzardi* (Nematoda: Filarioidea) and development of a PCR-based method for their detection in skin biopsies (vol 31, pg 169, 2001). Int J Parasitol. 2001;31(8):850–1.
152. Tang TH, Lopez-Velez R, Lanza M, Shelley AJ, Rubio JM, Luz SL. Nested PCR to detect and distinguish the sympatric filarial species *Onchocerca volvulus*, *Mansonella ozzardi* and Mansonella perstans in the Amazon Region. Memorias do Instituto Oswaldo Cruz. 2010;105(6):823–8.
153. Leroy S, Duperray C, Morand S. Flow cytometry for parasite nematode genome size measurement. Mol Biochem Parasitol. 2003;128(1):91–3.

Chapter 6
Application of Molecular Pathology to Cutaneous Melanocytic Lesions

Jonathan L. Curry, Michael T. Tetzlaff, Alexander J. Lazar and Victor G. Prieto

Introduction

Primary cutaneous melanoma is one of the most serious types of skin cancer and accounts for a majority of skin cancer-related deaths. The incidence of cutaneous melanoma continues to rise and the percentage of people with this disease has more than doubled in the past 30 years [1]. The estimated lifetime risk of an American developing invasive melanoma is currently 1 in 59 and is projected to be 1 in 50 by the year 2015 [2].

Evaluation of skin biopsies of melanocytic lesions accounts for approximately one fifth of all biopsies in a general dermatopathology practice [3]. Since the incidence of melanoma continues to rise and estimated number of biopsies required to detect melanoma is 1 out of 30 biopsies, histological evaluation of biopsies will continue to become a significant component of a dermatopathology practice [4]. Definitive morphologic distinction between benign and malignant melanocytic lesions by light microscopy is routinely achieved without the aid of ancillary tests. However, a subset of melanocytic lesions requires additional studies such as immunohistochemistry and other techniques, including FISH and comparative genomic hybridization (CGH) [5–7].

In the past several years, we have seen a tremendous improvement of our understanding of the molecular characteristics of melanocytic nevi and melanoma. High throughput genomic analysis has identified critical signaling pathways in melanoma tumorigenesis. One of the key oncogenic pathways in melanomagenesis involves the RAS/mitogen-activated protein kinase (MAPK), also termed as

J. L. Curry (✉) · M. T. Tetzlaff · A. J. Lazar · V. G. Prieto
Department of Pathology, The University of Texas: MD Anderson
Cancer Center, Houston, TX 77030, USA
e-mail: JLCurry@mdanderson.org

© Springer Science+Business Media New York 2015
V. G. Prieto (ed.), *Precision Molecular Pathology of Dermatologic Diseases,*
Molecular Pathology Library 9, DOI 10.1007/978-1-4939-2861-3_6

extracellular regulated kinase (ERK) pathway and the PI-3-Kinase/AKT pathways [8, 9]. Identification of aberrations in these pathways has furthered our understanding of relevant mechanisms of the cell signal pathways in melanomagenesis and led to the application of targeted agents in clinical trials.

This chapter examines the application of molecular pathology in melanocytic lesions of the skin. Key mutations in melanocytic nevi and melanomas are discussed as well as the application of molecular techniques (e.g., IHC, FISH, and CGH) to aid in distinguishing benign and malignant melanocytic neoplasms. Potential pitfalls in interpretation of some ancillary diagnostic techniques will also receive attention. Also we review the molecular signatures of melanoma now critical for assignment of targeted therapy to patients in routine care and clinical trials with comment on the emerging issues of skin toxicities associated with the targeted therapy for metastatic melanoma.

Cell Signaling Pathway in Nevogenesis and Melanomagenesis

Awareness of the cell signaling pathways operative in melanocytes has provided critical insights into the genetic alterations seen in melanocytic nevi and melanoma. In general, there are currently three cell-signaling pathways in melanocytes critical for their survival and proliferation which include: (1) MAPK/ERK, (2) phosphoinositide-3 kinase (PI3K)-AKT/PTEN, and (3) upstream signaling receptors such as KIT, melanocortin-1 receptor (MC1R), and glutamate receptor metabotropic (GRM3) receptor [10]. Activation of RAS via receptor tyrosine kinase initiates cell signaling through the MAPK and PI3K-AKT pathways promoting cell cycle progression and growth [11]. The AKT pathway can be activated by upstream receptor such as tyrosine kinase receptors, loss of PTEN, or less commonly, activating mutations of PIK3CA or AKT. The tyrosine kinase receptor for stem cell factor (SCF) encoded by *KIT* is critical for melanocyte migration and survival [12]. Activation of KIT targets the master regulator of melanocytes and microphthalmia transcription factor (MiTF). Phosphorylation of MiTF by ERK2 and p90RSK (p90 ribosomal S6 kinase) upon cKIT activation results its translocation to the nucleus and regulation of melanogenic protein tyrosinase (TYR), pro-survival protein BCL-2, and cell cycle protein p16INK4a [13, 14]. *MC1R,* a gene, is transmembrane G protein receptor expressed in melanocytes. The α-melanocyte stimulating hormone (α-MSH) binds to MC1R and stimulates adenylyl cyclase and increases cyclic adenosine monophosphate (cAMP) [15]. The α-MSH/MC1R pathway regulates melanin synthesis, melanocyte proliferation, and survival via transcriptional activation of MiTF, TYR, and other downstream targets [16, 17]. An emerging finding is that of activating mutations in the heterotrimeric G-protein coupled GRM3 receptor leading to downstream activation of the MEK and ERK pathway through phospholipase C (PLC) and protein kinase C (PKC). Additional study of this pathway is ongoing. Additional genes affected in cutaneous melanoma include *P16*, *CYCD1*, and *CDK4*, but like *MC1R* and *GRM3*, these are not yet associated with specific targeted therapy interventions, but do represent promising targets in a subset of melanomas.

Frequent Mutations in Melanocytic Nevi and Melanoma

Genetic Mutations in RAS

The *RAS oncogene* family includes *NRAS*, *HRAS*, and *KRAS*. Activated RAS recruits RAF which activates MEK and ERK and promotes cell proliferation, differentiation, and survival. *NRAS* isoforms have been associated with melanoma and congenital melanocytic nevi, and *HRAS* isoform is more commonly mutated in Spitz nevi. *KRAS* and *HRAS* mutations are infrequent in cutaneous melanoma [18]. *NRAS* mutations in melanocytic nevi and melanoma most commonly occur in exons 2 and 3 (previously known as exons 1 and 2, respectively). Congenital melanocytic nevi demonstrate the most prevalent *NRAS* mutations and approximately 65% of these mutations occur at codon 61 of exon 3 [19]. The most frequent mutations involve amino acid substitution of glutamine (Q) with lysine (K) or arginine (R) at position 61 (Q61K or Q61R) [20]. In contrast, melanocytic nevi with congenital pattern of growth typically will harbor *BRAF* and not *NRAS* mutation [21]. Cutaneous melanomas also harbor activating mutations in *NRAS* and similar to congenital nevi the frequent site of mutation is on codon 61 of exon 3 with Q61K or Q61R amino acid substitution. *NRAS* mutations occur in 14–20% of cutaneous melanoma; nodular and lentigo maligna histological subtypes are most frequently involved [22–24]. In contrast, alterations in *HRAS* are seen in nearly 30% of Spitz nevi [25, 26]. Increased copy number of chromosome 11p, the site of *HRAS* gene by CGH or FISH analysis has been reported in over 20% of Spitz nevi. Also mutations in *HRAS* can be seen in 29% of these lesions [27]. Analysis of 21 spitzoid melanomas failed to identify mutations in *HRAS*; thus, melanocytic lesions with histological features of Spitz and concurrent alterations in only *HRAS* gene (as detected by either mutation analysis or chromosomal amplification) may represent a molecular signature of Spitz nevi [26].

Genetic Mutations in RAF

RAF, a serine–threonine protein kinase, consists of three isoforms, ARAF, BRAF, and CRAF. RAF activation triggers MAPK signaling and cell proliferation via phosphorylation of downstream targets MEK and ERK. The N terminus of BRAF is constitutively activated in contrast to ARAF and CRAF, which require phosphorylation of the N terminus [28]. This distinction makes BRAF the primary isoform in the RAS/MAPK pathway and the isoform most susceptible for mutation in several solid tumors. The majority of *BRAF* mutations occur in exon 15 and involve a single

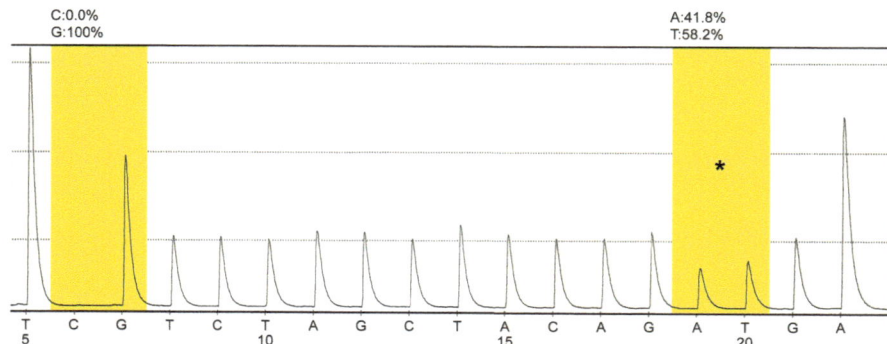

Fig. 6.1 Cutaneous melanoma with *BRAF V600E* mutation. Single point mutation involving DNA base substitution from thymine to adenine (T to A) (*) that converts amino acid valine (V) to glutamic acid (E) at the 600 amino acid position

point mutation with a DNA base substitution from thymine to adenine (T to A) that converts valine to glutamic acid at the 600th position of the amino acid (*BRAF V600E*; Fig. 6.1) and less frequently V600K, V600R, K601N, L597R, L597Q, G596R, and D594N [29]. Codons 595–600 from exon 15 are the most common mutation site for the *BRAF* gene followed by mutations codons 468–474 from exon 11. Compared with wild type BRAF, mutant *BRAF V600E* demonstrates an almost 500-fold increase in activity. Mutation in the *BRAF* gene located on chromosome 7 accounts for approximately 80 % of activation mutations in benign nevi and 50–60 % in primary cutaneous melanoma [30–32]. However, the presence of *BRAF* mutation in itself is not a marker of malignancy since such mutations are very frequent in benign melanocytic nevi. In fact, mutant *BRAF* in melanocytic nevi appears to induce senescence and growth arrest. Oncogene-induced *BRAF V600E* cellular senescence is a possible cellular mechanism in melanocytic nevi that allows benign nevi to become growth arrested and stable lesions for decades [33].

Typically, *NRAS* and *BRAF* mutations appear mutually exclusive; however, there are small percentages of melanomas that may harbor both *NRAS* and *BRAF* mutations (Fig. 6.2). In one study, double mutant *NRAS* and *BRAF* melanomas accounted for approximately 1.3 % of the cases analyzed [24, 34, 35]. On rare occasions melanomas may harbor combinations of other multiple mutations such as *NRAS* with *PIK3CA or CTNNB1* or *BRAF* with *PTEN, AKT1, or CTNNB1* [29].

Genetic Mutations in KIT

KIT is a tyrosine kinase growth factor receptor and *KIT* mutations and/or increased copy numbers are seen in acral lentiginous/mucosal melanomas and melanomas in skin with chronic sun damage (CSD) and ranges from 15 to 20 % of mutations in this type [36, 37]. Some studies did not reveal elevated instances of *KIT* mutations in CSD and additional studies are needed for clarification [38]. *KIT* mutation pro-

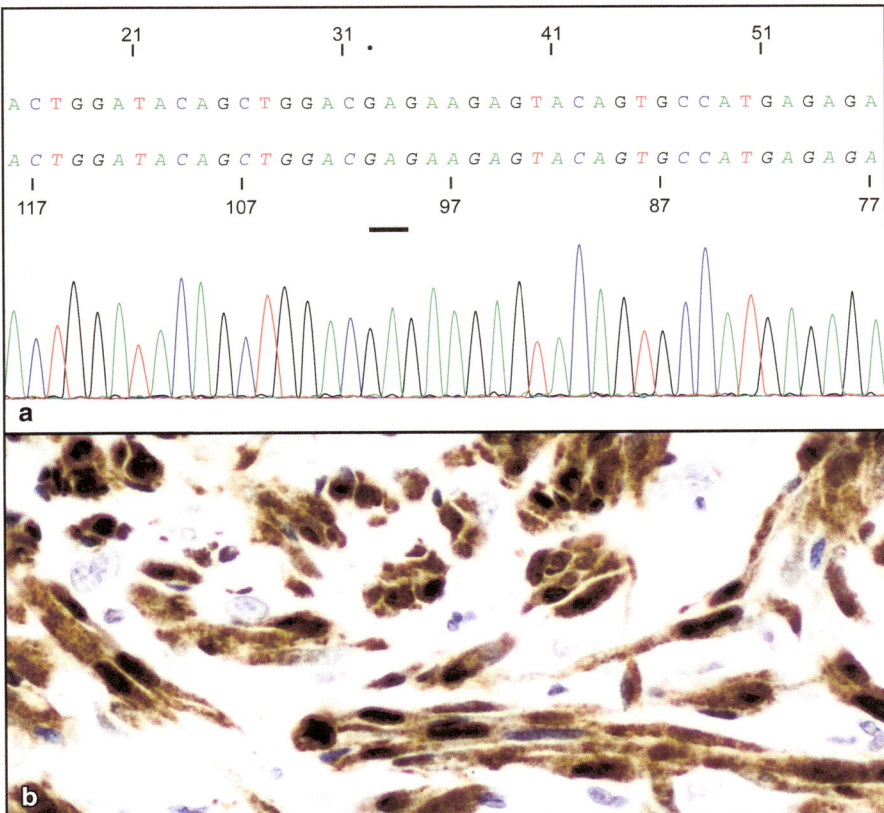

Fig. 6.2 Cutaneous melanoma with both *BRAF V600E* and *NRAS* Q61R mutations. A *BRAF V600E* point mutation was present, similar to Fig. 6.1 and in addition **a** Single point mutation involving DNA base substitution adenine to guanine (A to G) in codon 61 of *NRAS (bar)* gene that converts amino acid glutamine (Q) to arginine (R). **b** Invasive melanoma composed of nest of tumor cells with spindle shaped morphology. Tumor cells are reactive for S100 (nuclear and cytoplasmic reactivity)

motes ligand-independent *KIT* dimerization and constitutive activation of MAPK and PI3K-AKT pathways to promote proliferative and survival advantage for melanoma cells [39, 40]. Most mutations in *KIT* in melanomas occur on exon 11, which are also seen in gastrointestinal stromal tumor (GIST), but mutations in exons 13 and 17 are also relatively common in melanoma [41, 42]. Although, melanomas and GIST may demonstrate overlapping mutation spectra in *KIT*, there are distinct differences. The majority of exon 11 mutations in melanomas are substitution mutations in contrast to deletions or insertion mutations seen in GIST [43]. Exon 9 mutations are seen in up to 15 % of GIST but are infrequent in melanomas and increase in KIT copy number or amplification may occur in 30 % of a subset of melanomas while such findings are rarely observed in GIST [29, 44].

Genetic Mutations in GNAQ/GNA11

GNAQ and *GNA11* encode for the α-subunit of G-protein-coupled receptor. Mutations in *GNAQ* in melanocytic lesions exclusively occur at codon 209 with subsequent amino acid changes of glutamine to leucine or proline (Q209L or Q209P). GTP hydrolysis is prevented in mutant forms of *GNAQ*, thus resulting in a constitutive activation of this G-protein. A subset of benign and malignant melanocytic lesions harbor *GNAQ* mutations and similar to *BRAF* and *NRAS* mutations appear to be an early event in MAPK activation since mutations in *GNAQ* alone appear insufficient for melanomagenesis. *GNAQ* mutations have been detected in 83 % of blue nevi, 50 % of melanoma with blue nevus features, 46 % of uveal melanoma, and in 4 % of melanomas on chronically sun-damaged skin [45]. *GNA11* Q209 mutations occur in only 7 % of blue nevi. Similar percentages of *GNAQ* and *GNA11* mutations were observed in uveal melanomas, 46 and 32 %, respectively [46].

Molecular Platforms in Melanoma Mutation Analysis

Multiple sequencing molecular platforms are available to examine for *BRAF, NRAS, KIT, and GNAQ/GNA11* mutations in cutaneous melanomas. Sanger chain termination sequencing of amplified DNA (deoxyribonucleic acid) by polymerase chain reaction (PCR) led to the detection of *BRAF, NRAS, and KIT* mutations in cutaneous melanoma. Mutation analysis by Sanger sequencing provides complete sequence between the sequencing primer pairs and allows for the detection of DNA base pair substitutions, deletions, and insertions. Changes in chromosomal copy number and translocations cannot be detected by Sanger sequencing method [47]. Since recurrent mutations in melanomas appear to be clustered at particular genomic hot spots, pyrosequencing, allele-specific real-time polymerase chain reaction (RT-PCR), RT-PCR melting curve analysis, and mass spectroscopy-based mutation analysis allowed for faster, more sensitive methods in detection of predetermined hot spot mutations in cutaneous melanoma. Screening genes for nonrecurrent mutations in melanoma will require alternative molecular techniques and next generation sequencing platforms which will allow whole genome sequencing [47].

Of the known mutations to occur in cutaneous melanoma, *BRAF V600E* mutation appears to account for the highest percentage of mutations in cutaneous melanoma. The Cobas 4800 V600 mutation test by Roche is a Food and Drug Administration (FDA) approved in vitro diagnostic device for evaluation of *BRAF V600E* mutation in formalin-fixed paraffin-embedded tissue samples of melanoma. The sensitivity of detecting *BRAF V600E* by Cobas 4800 is reported to be greater than 99 % with a specificity of 88 % and the device is intended to identify patients who may benefit from therapy with selective *BRAF* inhibitor (BRAFi) vemurafenib [48].

Amplification of DNA by PCR remains central in evaluating for genomic mutations in melanoma. Melanin pigment is a known inhibitor of PCR and on occasion evaluation of tissue samples for mutation analysis may yield no results due to non-amplifiable DNA [49]. This may become an issue with melanomas that are heavily pigmented. One possible way to circumvent this problem is to repeat mutational analysis on tumor specimens from different blocks and/or different tissue sources from a patient if other material is available. Otherwise, there is a small subset of tumors where mutation analysis cannot be obtained despite repeat analysis and techniques to overcome melanin inhibition.

Dysplastic Nevus (DN) Syndrome and Familial Melanoma

The search for altered genes that could underlie the development of familial melanoma has directed investigations at the *CDKN2A/INK4A* gene on chromosome 9p21 which codes for a cyclin-dependent kinase inhibitor (CDKI) protein, p16INK4a [50]. The *CDKN2A/INK4A* gene is a major melanoma susceptibility locus associated with familial melanoma and dysplastic nevus (DN) syndrome or familial atypical multiple mole melanoma (FAMMM) [51–53]. The importance of tumor suppressors like p16INK4a as potential barriers to the development of melanoma has been illustrated in cell cultures and human tissue [54, 55]. Upregulation of p16INK4a was seen to inhibit normal melanocyte growth in culture and loss of replicative potential in melanocytic nevi [31, 33]. In a subset of patients, oncogene-induced cellular senescence appears to be an important barrier against further nevus growth and formation of cutaneous melanoma in a subset of patients.

Genetic alterations in acquired DN appear complex and include loss of tumor suppressor genes and altered function of oncogenes, housekeeping genes, growth factors, and extracellular matrix proteins. Molecular analyses have suggested that there may be alterations in the same set of susceptibility genes in DN and cutaneous melanoma. A thorough review of the molecular aspects of dysplastic nevi is available by Hussein et al [56]. In summary, dysplastic nevi may manifest from karyotypic alteration in chromosome 1p and 9p, allelic loss at chromosome 1p, 9p, and 17p, loss of tumor suppressor genes, *p16/CDKN2A* and *p53*, microsatellite instability, alterations in mismatch repair proteins, activation of B-raf, ras, and myc oncogenes, and alterations in extracellular matrix proteins (collagen type I, III, VI, tenascin, and fibronectin) and cytokines/growth factors [56].

Applications of Molecular Techniques in Diagnosis

Immunohistochemistry

The use of immunohistochemistry when evaluating melanocytic lesions may become necessary when the distinction between various types of benign melanocytic nevi and melanoma is not readily apparent upon examination of hematoxylin and eosin (H&E) stained sections. The standard antibodies used in dermatopathology

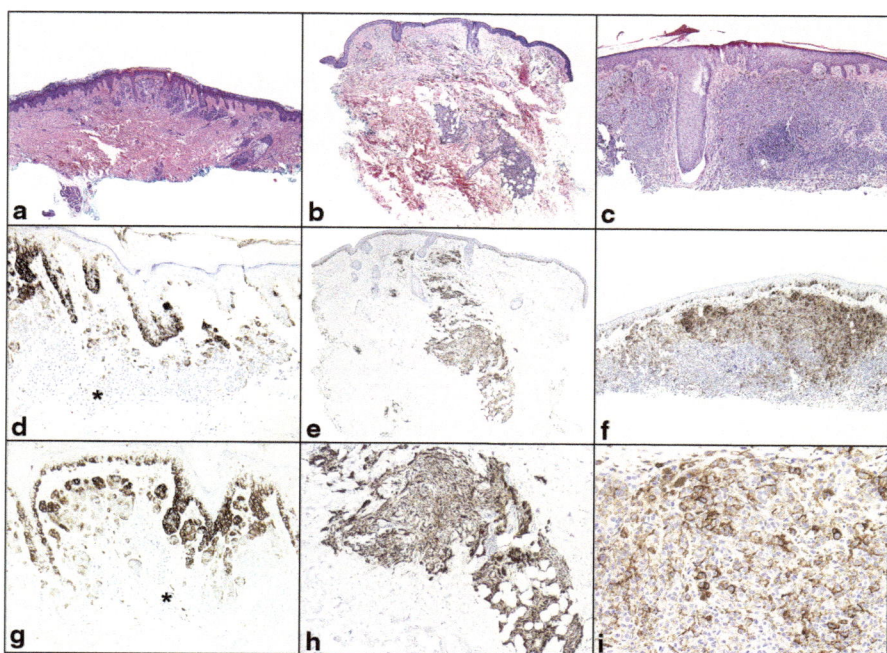

Fig. 6.3 Pattern of HMB-45 labeling in **a** melanocytic nevi, **b** Spitz nevi, and **c** invasive mela-noma. HMB-45 labels melanocytes in the epidermis and in the papillary dermis and superficial reticular dermis. **d** and **g** There is loss of HMB-45 labeling (normal maturation pattern in benign melanocytic nevi) with progressive descent into the deep reticular dermis (*). **e** and **h** Spitz nevi may demonstrate normal maturation pattern with respect to HMB-45 or a diffuse, uniform pattern of labeling. **f** and **i** Contrast to invasive melanoma with patchy labeling of HMB-45

practice for these types of lesions include S100, HMB-45 (anti-gp100), anti-MART-1, and *MIB1* (anti-Ki67) [57–59].

HMB-45 and anti-MART-1 label intraepidermal melanocytes and thus the extent of upward pagetoid upward migration of melanocytes in the epidermis may be high-lighted with either of these antibodies. Benign melanocytic nevi will demonstrate maturation sequence or loss of HMB-45 labeling with progressive descent into the dermis (Fig. 6.3). Exceptions to this pattern of labeling with HMB-45 in benign le-sions include blue nevi and subset of Spitz nevi. These two lesions may demonstrate a diffuse labeling pattern with respect to HMB-45 (Fig. 6.3). In contrast, melanomas will consistently demonstrate a patchy pattern of labeling with HMB-45 (Fig. 6.3).

Evaluation of the proliferative rate of the dermal component of melanocytic tu-mor is measured by Ki-67. This marker also aids in the distinction between benign and malignant melanocytic proliferations. Benign melanocytic nevi (ordinary, Spitz, and dysplastic) demonstrate less than 1–10 % labeling with *MIB1* (anti-Ki-67). However, melanomas demonstrated a proliferative rate up to 16.4 % with *MIB1* and absence of orderly pattern of labeling in the dermis [60]. Double labeling with MART-1 (cytoplasmic, red reactivity)/Ki-67 (nuclear, brown reactivity) enhances

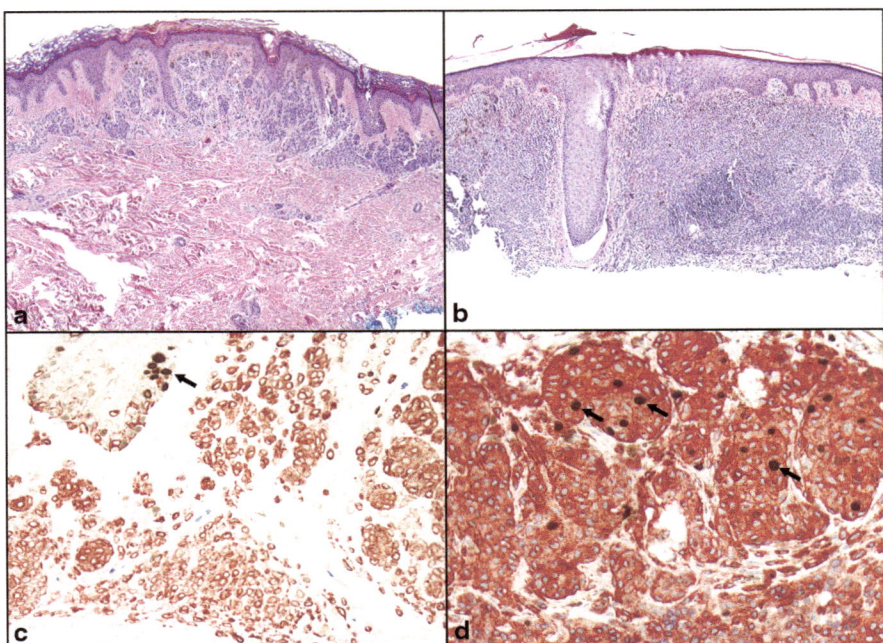

Fig. 6.4 Proliferative index of **a** melanocytic nevi and, **b** invasive melanoma with double stain Mart-1/Ki-67. **c** Melanocytic nevi demonstrate a low proliferative index of the dermal melanocytes (Mart-1 positive cells, *red*, cytoplasmic reactivity). The dermal melanocytes demonstrate absence of labeling with Ki-67 (*brown*, nuclear reactivity). Basal keratinocytes serve as a positive internal control for Ki-67 labeling *(arrow)*. **d** Invasive melanoma with increase proliferative rate with many Mart-1 (*red*, cytoplasmic labeling)/Ki-67 (*brown*, nuclear labeling) positive cells *(arrows)*

the evaluation of proliferative index in melanocytes, and is particularly useful in lesions with a high number of background lymphocytes (Fig. 6.4) [59].

Macrophages may be reactive with anti-MART-1 and may be interpreted as invasive melanoma cells [61]. Melanocytic nevi uniformly label with anti-MART-1 whereas desmoplastic melanoma may demonstrate weak, variable expression for MART-1 antibody.

Comparative Genomic Hybridization

Chromosomal abnormalities have been recognized in melanoma for decades [62–68]. The advent of CGH enabled a systematic characterization of melanoma at the genomic level. In traditional CGH, DNA derived from a tumor of interest is labeled with a discrete fluorochrome and mixed together with an equimolar amount of reference DNA labeled with a different fluorochrome. This mixture is hybridized onto denatured metaphase chromosomal spreads in the conventional method or onto an array containing serially arranged portions of DNA representing the entire genome in the array platform. Chromosomal gains in the tumor sample are represented by increased tumor-specific fluorochrome at a specific locus while losses in the tumor exhibit increased reference-specific fluorochrome at that site.

A critical development in our understanding of the pathogenesis of melanoma came from the work of Bastian and colleagues who initially utilized CGH to describe chromosomal gains and losses in primary melanomas from 32 patients [69]. They identified that primary melanomas were typified by multiple gains and losses in discrete regions of the genome. Subsequently, CGH was applied to a series of melanomas ($n = 132$) and melanocytic nevi ($n = 54$) to demonstrate a distinct pattern of chromosomal aberrations in melanomas not present in nevi. Whereas greater than 95 % of melanomas demonstrated some degree of chromosomal copy number aberration, only a rare subset of melanocytic nevi (13 %, all of which were Spitz nevi) demonstrated a single isolated gain of the entire short arm of chromosome 11—a change not seen in any of the melanomas analyzed [70]. Furthermore, central to the distinction between melanomas and nevi (of varying sorts) as demonstrated by CGH is the fact that melanomas contain gains and/or losses in partial regions of the chromosome, whereas when nevi contain alterations, they typically involve whole chromosomes or whole chromosomal arms. CGH not only distinguishes between melanomas and nevi, but also demonstrated discrete, reproducible differences among melanomas of varying subtypes. In a landmark study, Bastian and colleagues further used CGH to demonstrate that melanomas of varying subtypes (grouped according to whether they arose on or sites with or without chronic sun exposure) demonstrated distinct patterns of genomic alterations, including the frequency of oncogene mutations as well as differences in chromosomal aberrations. These findings argue that melanoma is a heterogeneous disease, arising through different mechanisms, which are a function—at least in part—of their anatomic location and the degree of antecedent ultraviolet light exposure [22].

Because CGH simultaneously scans the entire genome for all possible copy number alterations, it has considerable promise as a diagnostic tool in melanocytic tumors. However, there are many practical issues that limit the utility of CGH in a routine diagnostic setting. First, it requires a relatively large amount of pure tumor cells which can be difficult to obtain in some lesions and could compromise a thorough histopathologic assessment of a lesion. Lesions with relatively few tumor cells or lesions with a high degree of admixed inflammatory or stromal cells are also less amenable to CGH analysis because the DNA obtained from the non-tumoral cells can obscure the chromosomal abnormalities present in the background tumor cells. In addition, the abnormality must be present in a sufficient number of tumor cells to be detectable in the analysis. Finally, the DNA obtained must be suitable for subsequent enzymatic manipulations for fluorescent labeling reactions [71, 72].

Fluorescence In situ Hybridization

The limitations of conventional and array CGH necessitated the development of an assay that exploits the differences among melanocytic tumors described by CGH,

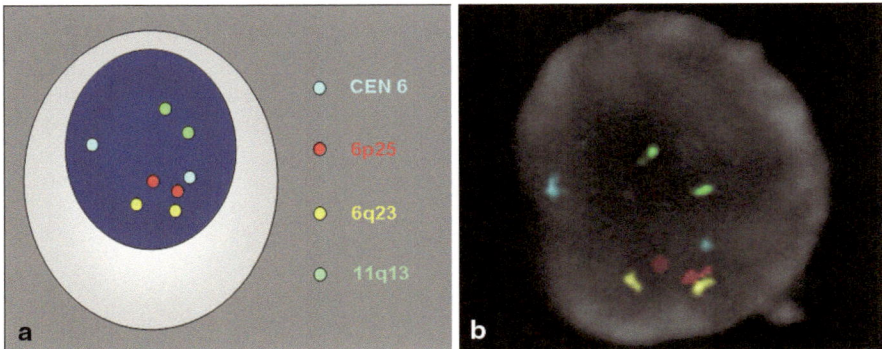

Fig. 6.5 Normal FISH analysis with four probe melanoma cocktail (*CEN* 6 = *aqua* dot, *RREB1* or 6p25 = *red* dot, *MYB* or 6q23 = *yellow* dot and *CCND1* or 11q13 = *green* dot). **a** cartoon, and **b** FISH of normal nuclei with two pairs of each probe is used in the four probe melanoma cocktail

but which is more amenable to routine clinical practice. FISH offers important advantages over CGH as a routine and practical clinical assay. FISH utilizes fluorescently labeled probes corresponding to discrete chromosomal locations that are hybridized to routine (5 µm) formalin fixed paraffin embedded tissue sections. The number of fluorescent signals per nucleus (described as "dots") is counted, and aberrations are described as a percentage of tumor nuclei carrying greater or fewer than two signals. FISH offers the ability to evaluate copy number aberrations at a cellular level and further, to correlate any changes in copy number at particular locus (corresponding to a specific fluorescent probe) with cellular morphology under conventional light microscopy.

The FISH assay for melanoma evolved directly from the CGH studies of Bastian and colleagues [73]. A retrospective analysis of the original CGH data from the series of 186 of primary melanomas and nevi identified 13 loci spanning 8 different chromosomes which in varying combinations best discriminated between melanomas and nevi. FISH probes corresponding to these regions were chosen and configured into different panels of probe combinations and applied to a series of melanomas and nevi to determine the optimum combination. Four probes were identified that appeared to yield the most effective distinction between melanomas and nevi: *RREB1* or 6p25 (red dot), *CEN6* or centromere 6 (aqua dot), *MYB* or 6q23 (yellow dot) and *CCND1* or 11q13 (green dot; Fig. 6.5). The centromere 6 probe is used to quantitate relative gains (or loss) of the other loci on this chromosome. Further studies generated the following algorithm that best discriminated between melanomas and nevi: (1) more than 38 % of the tumor nuclei contain greater than 2 signals for 11q13 or, (2) more than 29 % of tumor nuclei contain greater than 2 signals for 6p25 or, (3) more than 55 % of the tumor nuclei contain more 6p25 signals than centromere 6 signals, or (4) more than 40 % of the tumor nuclei contain fewer 6q23 signals than centromere 6 signals. Positivity for any of these parameters was determined as a positive test for melanoma. Numerous studies have subsequently tested the applicability of this FISH assay as a proof of principle in the distinc-

Table 6.1 Sensitivity and specificity of FISH in various types of melanocytic nevi and cutaneous melanoma

Lesion type	Melano-mas tested	Melanomas positive	Sensitiv-ity %	Nevi tested	Nevi negative	Speci-ficity %
Proof of principle [73, 74]	123	102	83	110	103	94
Ambiguous [85]	12	6	50	6	4	66
Proof of principle [75]	20	18	90	20	19	95
Lentiginous junctional melanoma of elderly [76]	19	16	84	19	19	100
Melanoma and nevus [76]	36	28	78	36	36	100
Blue nevus-like metas-tasis versus epithelioid blue nevus [78]	10	9	90	10	10	100
Metastatic melanoma versus intranodal nevus [79]	42	34	81	17	16	94
Superficial pagetoid melanocytosis [80]	7	5	71	6	6	100
Nevoid melanoma versus nevus [81]	10	10	100	10	10	100
Conjunctival melanoma versus nevus [82]	6	6	100	4	4	100
Desmoplastic mela-noma versus sclerosing nevi [83]	15	7	47	15	15	100
Blue nevus-like mela-noma versus cellular blue nevus [84]	5	5	100	12	12	100
Proof of principle [77]	20	17	85	19	17	90
Ambiguous [77]	21	9	43	69	55	80

tion between histopathologically unambiguous melanomas and nevi (Table 6.1) [74–77]. Additional studies have described the applicability of the FISH assay to different histopathological settings, including lentiginous junctional melanoma of the elderly [76]; blue nevus-like metastatic melanoma versus epithelioid blue nevus [78]; metastatic melanoma to lymph node versus intranodal nevus [79]; pagetoid melanocytosis as a distinctive subtype of melanoma [80]; nevoid melanoma versus benign melanocytic nevus [81]; conjunctival melanomas versus conjunctival nevi [82]; desmoplastic melanomas versus sclerosing melanocytic nevi [83]; and blue nevus-like melanoma versus cellular blue nevi [84]. From these preliminary studies, the overall sensitivity of FISH in distinguishing among melanomas and nevi of the indicated subtypes from various anatomic locations was ~80 % with an overall specificity of >90 %. However, it is important not to overestimate the value of FISH in a routine diagnostic setting since an important and often understated limitation inherent to the above studies was their reliance on histopathologically unambiguous melanomas and nevi to determine the utility of FISH. In morphologically unambiguous lesions, an experienced dermatopathologist would rarely—if ever—exclusively rely on a FISH assay for diagnostic purposes. An important question for the FISH assay thus became whether the FISH assay was applicable to histopathologically ambiguous lesions. In their original study, Gerami et al. applied the FISH assay to 27 ambiguous lesions—6 of which developed metastases and 21 of which were "event free" with a follow-up period of at least 5 years [73]. Of these cases, all 6 primary tumors that eventually developed metastases were FISH-positive, while only 6 of the 21 cases without metastases were FISH-positive. The latter observation was interpreted as melanomas that were either cured by excision or inadequately followed to detect their eventual metastases, while the former was interpreted as a high degree of sensitivity of FISH in identifying *bona fide* melanomas.

The applicability of FISH to ambiguous melanocytic tumors was further addressed in two important studies [77, 85]. Gaiser et al. applied the FISH assay to a series of 22 melanocytic tumors and compared the FISH results with histopathologic assessment, array CGH, and clinical follow up. Of seven cases with ambiguous histology but benign follow-up (range: 41–108 months), 2 cases yielded a positive FISH result; none of these was confirmed by array CGH. Of five cases with ambiguous histology but with malignant follow-up, three were positive by FISH, and two of these were confirmed by array CGH (CGH was not feasible for the third). Of the seven histopathologically unambiguous melanomas, three were FISH positive (one with malignant follow-up and two with 84 and 85 months, respectively, with benign follow-up), and for the one case in which it was feasible to do so, the FISH results were confirmed by array CGH. In contrast, two of the melanomas with negative follow-up (85 and 122 months of follow-up, respectively), and one of these was confirmed as negative by array CGH; two of the melanomas with malignant follow-up were also FISH negative, and notably, one of these cases demonstrated gains of 11q13 by array CGH. Overall, comparing FISH results with clinical outcome, there was a sensitivity of 60% and a specificity of 50% [85]. Similar observations were made by Vergier et al. who confirmed the utility of FISH in 43 unequivocal melanomas and nevi (85% sensitivity and 90% specificity) and then, compared the utility of expert histopathologic assessment to FISH in the characterization of 113 ambiguous tumors according to clinical outcome (grouped as either without recurrence or with metastases following a minimal 5 year follow-up) [77]. The latter analysis demonstrated that for the diagnosis of melanoma, expert histopathologic review yielded a sensitivity and specificity of 95 and 52%, respectively, while FISH yielded a sensitivity and specificity of only 43 and 80%, respectively. Of note, the combination of expert histopathologic review and FISH generated the optimum results, increasing the specificity of expert diagnosis alone to 76% and improving the sensitivity of FISH alone to 90% [77]. Their analysis further highlighted an important pitfall of FISH in the assessment of Spitz tumors where polyploidy is a well-described phenomenon [86]. The presence of polyploidy—additional, incremental copies of the entire genome rather than discrete regions—would potentially yield false positive FISH results (indicating a gain of 6p25 if not reviewed in the context of relative gains in *CEN6* probe and/or a gain of 11q13) in a FISH assay. Taken together, these studies underscore several important principles: (1) FISH is inadequate as a "stand alone" diagnostic assay in the differential diagnosis between melanoma and nevus, (2) a positive FISH test should not modify treatment in the absence of histopathologic confirmation, (3) a negative FISH test does not exclude melanoma if there is histopathologic evidence to support the diagnosis of melanoma, and (4) there are specific clinical-pathologic contexts in which FISH should be applied with caution, including desmoplastic/sclerotic lesions as well as Spitzoid lesions. The recommendation based on the findings of Vergier et al. is that the combination of FISH and expert histopathologic review yielded the highest combination of sensitivity and specificity [77].

Applications of Molecular Techniques in Targeted Therapy

Molecular Signature of Melanoma

Distinct subsets of cutaneous melanoma will harbor mutations in *BRAF, KIT, and NRAS*. The molecular disease model for melanoma allows further classification of tumors defined by the role(s) of key oncogene or tumor suppressor genes [87]. Alteration in the *RAS/RAF/MEK/ERK* cell signal pathway and constitutive activation of MAPK have been detected in nearly 80 % of cutaneous melanoma [88]. Mutational analysis of melanoma may not only provide prognostic information in a subset of patients but also be critical for treatment of advance stage disease with small molecular inhibitors and enrolment in clinical trials. Patients with *NRAS* mutations tend to demonstrate increased tumor thickness, which may correspond to the higher frequency of mutant *NRAS* in nodular subtypes of cutaneous melanomas which tend to greater, thicker tumors at initial biopsy. There was a trend to shorter melanoma specific survival and disease free survival in *NRAS* mutant melanomas [89]. The presence of mutant *BRAF* does not appear to have an effect on disease free interval (DFI) or overall survival (OS) [90]. However, it appears to impact OS after the diagnosis of distant metastasis or stage IV disease [35, 90]. Furthermore, patients with *BRAF* or *NRAS* mutations may develop central nervous system metastasis when compared to patients with wild-type tumors. Furthermore, the presence of *NRAS* mutation was an independent predictor of decreased survival in stage IV melanoma patients [35].

Small molecule inhibitors including imatinib, sorafenib, and dasatinib have targeted melanomas with mutated *KIT* and *BRAF*. *KIT* mutated tumors demonstrated a dramatic clinical responses in a subset of patients treated with imatinib with two complete responses, two durable partial responses, and two transient partial responses in 25 of the patients evaluated [91]. Several BRAF-selective inhibitors or second generation BRAFi have entered clinical trials. Vemurafenib (also known as PLX4032, RO5185426) is a selective BRAFi used in the treatment of advanced melanoma. A response rate of 81 % in 32 BRAF-mutated melanoma patients was reported in the phase I extension cohort [48]. Other second generation BRAF-selective inhibitor has already shown promising anti-tumor activity in the phase I study. Although, vemurafenib and other selective BRAFi may induce tumor response in patients with *BRAF* mutant melanoma, the duration of response generally ranges from two to greater than 18 months until acquired resistance to therapy develops, though occasionally more durable responses can be seen [48, 92].

Dermatologic toxicities are common in patients receiving targeted molecular inhibitors. Common skin toxicities associated with targeted therapy for the treatment of advanced stage melanoma include mild to moderate skin eruptions, sun sensitivity, fatigue, arthralgia, and squamous proliferations including keratosis pilaris, actinic keratosis, warty papules, keratoacanthomas (KA), and invasive squamous cell carcinomas [93–95]. As new small molecule inhibitors enter clinical trials, awareness of skin associated toxicities and the era of oncodermatopathology will become an important component of academic and community dermatopathology practices.

Summary and Conclusions

The field of melanoma research has identified unique sets of chromosomal abnormalities by CGH and FISH and recurring *BRAF*, *NRAS*, and *KIT* mutations by sequence analysis of certain subtypes of cutaneous melanoma. These molecular attributes of melanoma has had clinical applications in diagnosis, prognosis, and treatment. FISH analysis, when combined with clinical, morphologic, and IHC features has improved the sensitivity and specificity of detection of melanoma is a subset of melanocytic tumors. Evaluation of distinct mutations in melanoma has been critical for prognosis and identification of patients that may benefit from targeted therapy. Molecular testing of cutaneous melanoma for selection of targeted therapy and clinical trials has become routine practice in patient care in academic institutions and in the community settings.

Case Example

To demonstrate many of the principles described in the current chapter, we describe a case in which we present the morphologic parameters of a challenging melanocytic tumor. We then demonstrate the application of both immunohistochemical and molecular FISH studies to further characterize the lesion to demonstrate how these various findings can be integrated into a diagnosis that directs the most appropriate management of the patient.

The case is one which we received in consultation: A shave biopsy specimen from the right buttock of a 13-year-old girl. Low power examination reveals an asymmetric predominantly intradermal melanocytic proliferation with an asymmetric lymphohistiocytic inflammatory host response. Higher power examination reveals the lesion to be comprised predominantly of epithelioid cells with pleomorphic, oval nuclei, and prominent nucleoli. Multinucleated forms and mitotic figures are also noted, and there is the minimal maturation with dermal descent (Fig. 6.6)

IHC studies were performed. Antibodies for HMB-45 antigen demonstrate patchy reactivity throughout the lesion. Furthermore, double labeling with a MART-1/Ki-67 cocktail reveals an increased proliferative index in the dermal melanocytes

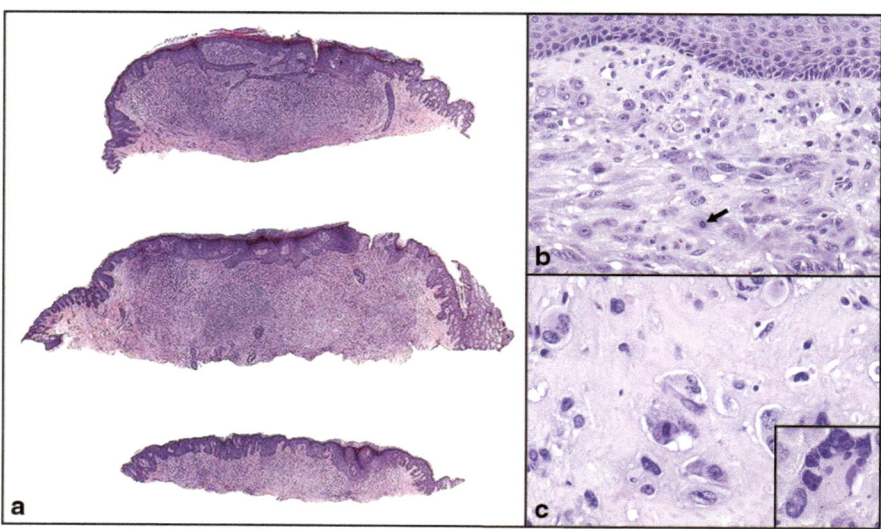

Fig. 6.6 Right buttock lesion of a 13-year-old girl. **a** Asymmetric predominantly intradermal atypical melanocytic proliferation (Fig. 6.6). **b** Epithelioid cells in dermis with minimal maturation with progressive descent and scattered mitoses *(arrow)*. **c** Tumor cells are pleomorphic multinucleated forms *(inset)* and abundant eosinophilic cytoplasm, oval nuclei, prominent nucleoli, and minimal maturation with dermal descent

of ~10 %. In addition, there is apparently patchy reactivity in the melanocytes with antibodies for MART-1 (Fig. 6.7). Together with the morphologic findings, we favored a diagnosis of invasive melanoma.

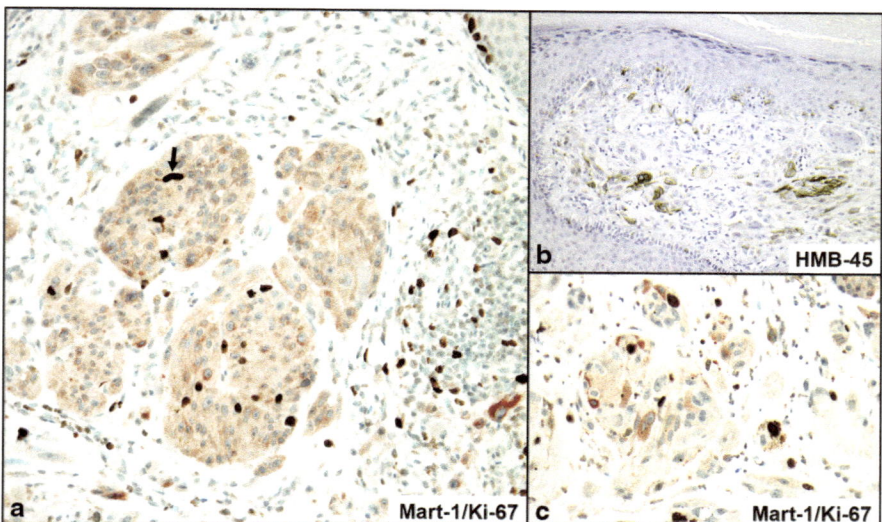

Fig. 6.7 Immunohistochemcial stains with Mart-1/Ki67 and HMB-45. **a** Increased proliferative index in the dermal melanocytes with double stain Mart-1 (*red*, cytoplasmic reactivity) and Ki-67 (*brown*, nuclear reactivity; *arrows*). **b** and **c** Patchy reactivity of neoplastic cells in the dermis with respect to HMB45 and Mart-1

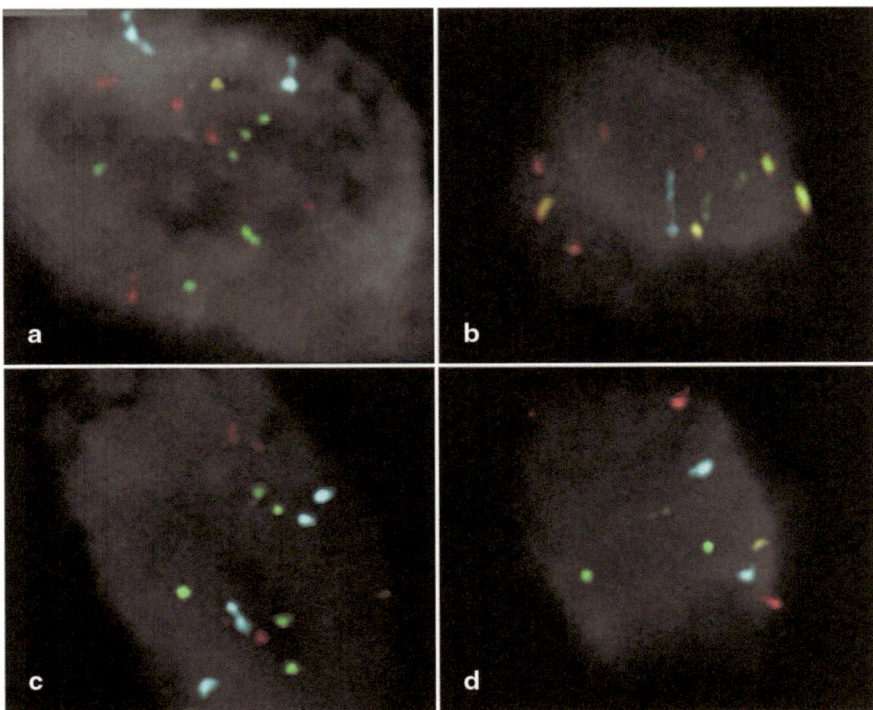

Fig. 6.8 FISH testing of melanocytic lesion detected nuclei with three chromosomal abnormalities patterns involving *RREB1* or 6p25 *(red dot)*, *MYB* or 6q23 *(gold dot)*:*CEN 6 (aqua dot)* ratio, and *CCND1* or 11q13 *(green dot)*. **a** and **b** Increased in *RREB1 (red dots)* and **c** *CCND1 (green dots)*. **c** and **d** Decreased in *MYB:Cen 6* (gold dots:aqua dots) ratio

To characterize the lesion further, we also submitted the lesion for FISH testing. FISH testing detected three chromosomal abnormalities involving *RREB1* (6p25), *MYB:CEN6* (6q23:CEN6) ratio, and *CCND1* (11q13). The other probe set, *RREB1:CEN6* (red:aqua) ratio, exhibited a signal pattern within the normal range. As shown in Fig. 6.8, approximately 35.64 % of the cells showed increased *RREB1* (red) signals (normal cut-off value < 16 %). Furthermore, approximately 48.51 % of the cells showed a decreased *MYB:CEN6* (gold:aqua) ratio (normal cutoff value < 42 %). Finally, approximately 33.66 % of the cells showed increased *CCND1* (green) signals (normal cut-off value < 19 %).

Together with the morphologic and IHC findings, these data supported the diagnosis of invasive melanoma.

References

1. Rigel DS. Epidemiology of melanoma. Semin Cutan Med Surg. 2010;29(4):204–9.
2. Jemal A, Siegel R, Ward E, Hao Y, Xu J, Thun MJ. Cancer statistics, 2009. CA Cancer J Clin. 2009;59(4):225–49.
3. Green AR, Elgart GW, Ma F, Federman DG, Kirsner RS. Documenting dermatology practice: ratio of cutaneous tumors biopsied that are malignant. Dermatol Surg. 2004;30(9):1208–9.
4. Hansen C, Wilkinson D, Hansen M, Argenziano G. How good are skin cancer clinics at melanoma detection? Number needed to treat variability across a national clinic group in Australia. J Am Acad Dermatol. 2009;61(4):599–604.
5. Zembowicz A, Prieto VG. Melanocytic lesions: current state of knowledge. Arch Pathol Lab Med. 2010;134(12):1738–39.
6. Zembowicz A, Prieto VG. Melanocytic lesions: current state of knowledge? Part II. Arch Pathol Lab Med. 2011;135(3):298–9.
7. Zembowicz A, Prieto VG. Melanocytic lesions: current state of knowledge–part III. Arch Pathol Lab Med. 2011;135(7):824.
8. Ibrahim N, Haluska FG. Molecular pathogenesis of cutaneous melanocytic neoplasms. Annu Rev Pathol. 2009;4:551–79.
9. Ko JM, Fisher DE. A new era: melanoma genetics and therapeutics. J Pathol. 2011;223(2): 241–50.
10. Prickett TD, Wei X, Cardenas-Navia I, et al. Exon capture analysis of G protein-coupled receptors identifies activating mutations in GRM3 in melanoma. Nat Genet. 2011;43(11):1119–26.
11. Vojtek AB, Hollenberg SM, Cooper JA. Mammalian Ras interacts directly with the serine/threonine kinase Raf. Cell. 1993;74(1):205–14.
12. Alexeev V, Yoon K. Distinctive role of the cKit receptor tyrosine kinase signaling in mammalian melanocytes. J Invest Dermatol. 2006;126(5):1102–10.
13. McGill GG, Horstmann M, Widlund HR, et al. Bcl2 regulation by the melanocyte master regulator Mitf modulates lineage survival and melanoma cell viability. Cell. 2002;109(6):707–18.
14. Loercher AE, Tank EM, Delston RB, Harbour JW. MITF links differentiation with cell cycle arrest in melanocytes by transcriptional activation of INK4A. J Cell Biol. 2005;168(1):35–40.
15. Mas JS, Gerritsen I, Hahmann C, Jimenez-Cervantes C, Garcia-Borron JC. Rate limiting factors in melanocortin 1 receptor signalling through the cAMP pathway. Pigment Cell Res. 2003;16(5):540–7.
16. Schaffer JV, Bolognia JL. The melanocortin-1 receptor: red hair and beyond. Arch Dermatol. 2001;137(11):1477–85.
17. Kadekaro AL, Kanto H, Kavanagh R, Abdel-Malek ZA. Significance of the melanocortin 1 receptor in regulating human melanocyte pigmentation, proliferation, and survival. Ann N Y Acad Sci. 2003;994:359–65.
18. Whitwam T, Vanbrocklin MW, Russo ME, et al. Differential oncogenic potential of activated RAS isoforms in melanocytes. Oncogene. 2007;26(31):4563–70.
19. Ross AL, Sanchez MI, Grichnik JM. Molecular nevogenesis. Dermatology research and practice. 2011:463184.
20. Takata M, Saida T. Genetic alterations in melanocytic tumors. J Dermatol Sci. 2006;43(1): 1–10.
21. Bauer J, Curtin JA, Pinkel D, Bastian BC. Congenital melanocytic nevi frequently harbor NRAS mutations but no BRAF mutations. J Invest Dermatol. 2007;127(1):179–82.
22. Curtin JA, Fridlyand J, Kageshita T, et al. Distinct sets of genetic alterations in melanoma. N Engl J Med. 2005;353(20):2135–47.
23. Lee JH, Choi JW, Kim YS. Frequencies of BRAF and NRAS mutations are different in histological types and sites of origin of cutaneous melanoma: a meta-analysis. Br J Dermatol. 2011;164(4):776–84.

24. Goel VK, Lazar AJ, Warneke CL, Redston MS, Haluska FG. Examination of mutations in BRAF, NRAS, and PTEN in primary cutaneous melanoma. J Invest Dermatol. 2006;126(1):154–60.
25. Bastian BC, LeBoit PE, Pinkel D. Mutations and copy number increase of HRAS in Spitz nevi with distinctive histopathological features. Am J Pathol. 2000;157(3):967–72.
26. Forno PD D, Pringle JH, Fletcher A, et al. BRAF, NRAS and HRAS mutations in spitzoid tumours and their possible pathogenetic significance. Br J Dermatol. 2009;161(2):364–72.
27. van Dijk MC, Bernsen MR, Ruiter DJ. Analysis of mutations in B-RAF, N-RAS, and H-RAS genes in the differential diagnosis of Spitz nevus and spitzoid melanoma. Am J Surg Pathol. 2005;29(9):1145–51.
28. Mason CS, Springer CJ, Cooper RG, Superti-Furga G, Marshall CJ, Marais R. Serine and tyrosine phosphorylations cooperate in Raf-1, but not B-Raf activation. EMBO J. 1999;18(8):2137–48.
29. Beadling C, Jacobson-Dunlop E, Hodi FS, et al. KIT gene mutations and copy number in melanoma subtypes. Clin Cancer Res. 2008;14(21):6821–8.
30. Davies H, Bignell GR, Cox C, et al. Mutations of the BRAF gene in human cancer. Nature. 2002;417(6892):949–54.
31. Pollock PM, Harper UL, Hansen KS, et al. High frequency of BRAF mutations in nevi. Nat Genet. 2003;33(1):19–20.
32. Hocker T, Tsao H. Ultraviolet radiation and melanoma: a systematic review and analysis of reported sequence variants. Hum Mutat. 2007;28(6):578–88.
33. Michaloglou C, Vredeveld LC, Soengas MS, et al. BRAFE600-associated senescence-like cell cycle arrest of human naevi. Nature. 2005;436(7051):720–4.
34. Ellerhorst JA, Greene VR, Ekmekcioglu S, et al. Clinical correlates of NRAS and BRAF mutations in primary human melanoma. Clin Cancer Res. 2011;17(2):229–35.
35. Jakob JA, Bassett RL, Ng CS, Lazar AF, Joseph RW, Alvarado GC, Rohlfs ML, Richard J, Curry JL, Gershenwald JE, Hwu P, Kim KB, Davies MA. NRAS Mutation Status is an Independent Prognostic Factor in Metastatic Melanoma. Cancer. 2012;118(16):4014–23.
36. Curtin JA, Busam K, Pinkel D, Bastian BC. Somatic activation of KIT in distinct subtypes of melanoma. J Clin Oncol. 2006;24(26):4340–6.
37. Torres-Cabala CA, Wang WL, Trent J, et al. Correlation between KIT expression and KIT mutation in melanoma: a study of 173 cases with emphasis on the acral-lentiginous/mucosal type. Mod Pathol. 2009;22(11):1446–56.
38. Handolias D, Salemi R, Murray W, et al. Mutations in KIT occur at low frequency in melanomas arising from anatomical sites associated with chronic and intermittent sun exposure. Pigment Cell Melanoma Res. 2010;23(2):210–5.
39. Liang R, Wallace AR, Schadendorf D, Rubin BP. The phosphatidyl inositol 3-kinase pathway is central to the pathogenesis of Kit-activated melanoma. Pigment Cell Melanoma Res. 2011;24(4):714–23.
40. Garrido MC, Bastian BC. KIT as a therapeutic target in melanoma. J Invest Dermatol. 2010;130(1):20–7.
41. Hornick JL, Fletcher CD. The role of KIT in the management of patients with gastrointestinal stromal tumors. Hum Pathol. 2007;38(5):679–87.
42. Corless CL, Heinrich MC. Molecular pathobiology of gastrointestinal stromal sarcomas. Annu Rev Pathol. 2008;3:557–86.
43. Woodman SE, Davies MA. Targeting KIT in melanoma: a paradigm of molecular medicine and targeted therapeutics. Biochem Pharmacol. 2010;80(5):568–74.
44. Ashida A, Takata M, Murata H, Kido K, Saida T. Pathological activation of KIT in metastatic tumors of acral and mucosal melanomas. Int J Cancer. 2009;124(4):862–8.
45. Van Raamsdonk CD, Bezrookove V, Green G, et al. Frequent somatic mutations of GNAQ in uveal melanoma and blue naevi. Nature. 2009;457(7229):599–602.
46. Van Raamsdonk CD, Griewank KG, Crosby MB, et al. Mutations in GNA11 in uveal melanoma. N Engl J Med. 2010;363(23):2191–9.

47. Ross JS, Cronin M. Whole cancer genome sequencing by next-generation methods. Am J Clin Pathol. 2011;136(4):527–39.
48. Chapman PB, Hauschild A, Robert C, et al. Improved survival with vemurafenib in melanoma with BRAF V600E mutation. N Engl J Med. 2011;364(26):2507–16.
49. Opel KL, Chung D, McCord BR. A study of PCR inhibition mechanisms using real time PCR. J Forensic Sci. 2010;55(1):25–33.
50. Haluska FG, Housman DE. Recent advances in the molecular genetics of malignant melanoma. Cancer Surv. 1995;25:277–92.
51. Czajkowski R, Placek W, Drewa G, Czajkowska A, Uchanska G. FAMMM syndrome: pathogenesis and management. Dermatol Surg. 2004;30(2 Pt 2):291–6.
52. Piepkorn M Melanoma genetics: an update with focus on the CDKN2A(p16)/ARF tumor suppressors. J Am Acad Dermatol. 2000;42(5 Pt 1):705–722; quiz 723–706.
53. Ranade K, Hussussian CJ, Sikorski RS, et al. Mutations associated with familial melanoma impair p16INK4 function. Nat Genet. 1995;10(1):114–6.
54. Sviderskaya EV, Hill SP, Evans-Whipp TJ, et al. p16(Ink4a) in melanocyte senescence and differentiation. J Natl Cancer Inst. 2002;94(6):446–54.
55. Gray-Schopfer VC, Cheong SC, Chong H, et al. Cellular senescence in naevi and immortalisation in melanoma: a role for p16? Br J Cancer. 2006;95(4):496–505.
56. Hussein MRWG. Molecular aspects of melanocytic dysplastic nevi. J Mol Diagn. 2002;4(2):9.
57. Ivan D, Prieto VG. Use of immunohistochemistry in the diagnosis of melanocytic lesions: applications and pitfalls. Future Oncol. 2010;6(7):1163–75.
58. Prieto VG, Shea CR. Use of immunohistochemistry in melanocytic lesions. J Cutan Pathol. 2008;35 Suppl 2:1–10.
59. Prieto VG, Shea CR. Immunohistochemistry of melanocytic proliferations. Arch Pathol Lab Med. 2011;135(7):853–9.
60. Rudolph P, Schubert C, Schubert B, Parwaresch R. Proliferation marker Ki-S5 as a diagnostic tool in melanocytic lesions. J Am Acad Dermatol. 1997;37(2 Pt 1):169–78.
61. Trejo O, Reed JA, Prieto VG. Atypical cells in human cutaneous re-excision scars for melanoma express p75NGFR, C56/N-CAM and GAP-43: evidence of early Schwann cell differentiation. J Cutan Pathol. 2002;29(7):397–406.
62. Balaban G, Herlyn M, Guerry Dt, et al. Cytogenetics of human malignant melanoma and premalignant lesions. Cancer Genet Cytogenet. 1984;11(4):429–39.
63. D'Alessandro I, Zitzelsberger H, Hutzler P, et al. Numerical aberrations of chromosome 7 detected in 15 microns paraffin-embedded tissue sections of primary cutaneous melanomas by fluorescence in situ hybridization and confocal laser scanning microscopy. J Cutan Pathol. 1997;24(2):70–5.
64. Isshiki K, Elder DE, Guerry D, Linnenbach AJ. Chromosome 10 allelic loss in malignant melanoma. Genes Chromosom Cancer. 1993;8(3):178–84.
65. Isshiki K, Seng BA, Elder DE, Guerry D, Linnenbach AJ. Chromosome 9 deletion in sporadic and familial melanomas in vivo. Oncogene. 1994;9(6):1649–53.
66. Millikin D, Meese E, Vogelstein B, Witkowski C, Trent J. Loss of heterozygosity for loci on the long arm of chromosome 6 in human malignant melanoma. Cancer Res. 1991;51(20):5449–53.
67. Thompson FH, Emerson J, Olson S, et al. Cytogenetics of 158 patients with regional or disseminated melanoma. Subset analysis of near-diploid and simple karyotypes. Cancer Genet Cytogenet. 1995;83(2):93–104.
68. Wolfe KQ, Southern SA, Herrington CS. Interphase cytogenetic demonstration of chromosome 9 loss in thick melanomas. J Cutan Pathol. 1997;24(7):398–402.
69. Bastian BC, LeBoit PE, Hamm H, Brocker EB, Pinkel D. Chromosomal gains and losses in primary cutaneous melanomas detected by comparative genomic hybridization. Cancer Res. 1998;58(10):2170–75.
70. Bastian BC, Olshen AB, LeBoit PE, Pinkel D. Classifying melanocytic tumors based on DNA copy number changes. Am J Pathol. 2003;163(5):1765–70.
71. Gerami P, Zembowicz A. Update on fluorescence in situ hybridization in melanoma: state of the art. Arch Pathol Lab Med. 2011;135(7):830–7.

72. Song J, Mooi WJ, Petronic-Rosic V, Shea CR, Stricker T, Krausz T. Nevus versus melanoma: to FISH, or not to FISH. Adv Anat Pathol. 2011;18(3):229–34.
73. Gerami P, Jewell SS, Morrison LE, et al. Fluorescence in situ hybridization (FISH) as an ancillary diagnostic tool in the diagnosis of melanoma. Am J Surg Pathol. 2009;33(8):1146–56.
74. Gerami P, Mafee M, Lurtsbarapa T, Guitart J, Haghighat Z, Newman M. Sensitivity of fluorescence in situ hybridization for melanoma diagnosis using *RREB1*, *MYB*, Cep6, and 11q13 probes in melanoma subtypes. Arch Dermatol. 2010;146(3):273–8.
75. Morey AL, Murali R, McCarthy SW, Mann GJ, Scolyer RA. Diagnosis of cutaneous melanocytic tumours by four-colour fluorescence in situ hybridisation. Pathology. 2009;41(4):383–7.
76. Newman MD, Mirzabeigi M, Gerami P. Chromosomal copy number changes supporting the classification of lentiginous junctional melanoma of the elderly as a subtype of melanoma. Mod Pathol. 2009;22(9):1258–62.
77. Vergier B, Prochazkova-Carlotti M, de la Fouchardiere A, et al. Fluorescence in situ hybridization, a diagnostic aid in ambiguous melanocytic tumors: European study of 113 cases. Mod Pathol. 2011;24(5):613–23.
78. Pouryazdanparast P, Newman M, Mafee M, Haghighat Z, Guitart J, Gerami P. Distinguishing epithelioid blue nevus from blue nevus-like cutaneous melanoma metastasis using fluorescence in situ hybridization. Am J Surg Pathol. 2009;33(9):1396–400.
79. Dalton SR, Gerami P, Kolaitis NA, et al. Use of fluorescence in situ hybridization (FISH) to distinguish intranodal nevus from metastatic melanoma. Am J Surg Pathol. 2010;34(2):231–7.
80. Gerami P, Barnhill RL, Beilfuss BA, LeBoit P, Schneider P, Guitart J. Superficial melanocytic neoplasms with pagetoid melanocytosis: a study of interobserver concordance and correlation with FISH. Am J Surg Pathol. 2010;34(6):816–21.
81. Gerami P, Wass A, Mafee M, Fang Y, Pulitzer MP, Busam KJ. Fluorescence in situ hybridization for distinguishing nevoid melanomas from mitotically active nevi. Am J Surg Pathol. 2009;33(12):1783–8.
82. Busam KJ, Fang Y, Jhanwar SC, Pulitzer MP, Marr B, Abramson DH. Distinction of conjunctival melanocytic nevi from melanomas by fluorescence in situ hybridization. J Cutan Pathol. 2010;37(2):196–203.
83. Gerami P, Beilfuss B, Haghighat Z, Fang Y, Jhanwar S, Busam KJ. Fluorescence in situ hybridization as an ancillary method for the distinction of desmoplastic melanomas from sclerosing melanocytic nevi. J Cutan Pathol. 2011;38(4):329–34.
84. Gammon B, Beilfuss B, Guitart J, Busam KJ, Gerami P. Fluorescence in situ hybridization for distinguishing cellular blue nevi from blue nevus-like melanoma. J Cutan Pathol. 2011;38(4):335–41.
85. Gaiser T, Kutzner H, Palmedo G, et al. Classifying ambiguous melanocytic lesions with FISH and correlation with clinical long-term follow up. Mod Pathol. 2010;23(3):413–9.
86. Isaac AK, Lertsburapa T, Pathria Mundi J, Martini M, Guitart J, Gerami P. Polyploidy in Spitz nevi: a not uncommon karyotypic abnormality identifiable by fluorescence in situ hybridization. Am J Dermatopathol. 2010;32(2):144–8.
87. Vidwans SJ, Flaherty KT, Fisher DE, Tenenbaum JM, Travers MD, Shrager J. A melanoma molecular disease model. PLoS ONE. 2011;6(3):e18257.
88. Gaudi S, Messina JL. Molecular bases of cutaneous and uveal melanomas. Patholog Res Int. 2011;2011:159421.
89. Devitt B, Liu W, Salemi R, et al. Clinical outcome and pathological features associated with NRAS mutation in cutaneous melanoma. Pigment Cell Melanoma Res. 2011;24(4):666–672.
90. Long GV, Menzies AM, Nagrial AM, et al. Prognostic and clinicopathologic associations of oncogenic BRAF in metastatic melanoma. J Clin Oncol. 2011;29(10):1239–46.
91. Carvajal RD, Antonescu CR, Wolchok JD, et al. KIT as a therapeutic target in metastatic melanoma. JAMA. 2011;305(22):2327–34.
92. Flaherty KT, Puzanov I, Kim KB, et al. Inhibition of mutated, activated BRAF in metastatic melanoma. N Engl J Med. 2010;363(9):809–19.
93. Kwon EJ, Kish LS, Jaworsky C. The histologic spectrum of epithelial neoplasms induced by sorafenib. J Am Acad Dermatol. 2009;61(3):522–7.

94. Smith KJ, Haley H, Hamza S, Skelton HG. Eruptive keratoacanthoma-type squamous cell carcinomas in patients taking sorafenib for the treatment of solid tumors. Dermatol Surg. 2009;35(11):1766–70.
95. Dubauskas Z, Kunishige J, Prieto VG, Jonasch E, Hwu P, Tannir NM. Cutaneous squamous cell carcinoma and inflammation of actinic keratoses associated with sorafenib. Clin Genitourin Cancer. 2009;7(1):20–3.

Chapter 7
Application of Molecular Pathology to Tissue Identification in Cutaneous Pathology

Michael T. Tetzlaff, Jonathan L. Curry and Victor G. Prieto

Introduction

Misidentification of pathologic samples remains a minor but critically important and potentially devastating source of both medical error and subsequent litigation in pathology practices. Large-scale studies have estimated such "biopsy misidentification" errors at a frequency ranging from 0.25 to 0.4 % [1–3]. In the case of small biopsy specimens, such errors can have profound consequences for subsequent patient management decisions insofar as those decisions are directly impacted by the results of the biopsy interpretation [2].

An analogous "identity crisis" occurs in patients, who develop graft versus host disease (GVHD) following stem cell transplantation, solid organ transplantation and transfusion [4]. In these clinical contexts, exogenously derived immunocompetent T lymphocytes stage an immunologic response against foreign recipient tissues. This attack elicits an array of characteristic clinicopathologic features, including a skin rash (typically a maculopapular erythematous rash involving the trunk and extremities), hepatic dysfunction (manifested principally by an elevated total serum bilirubin and alkaline phosphatase), and intestinal upset (typically manifested by pain, nausea/vomiting, and/or diarrhea). GVHD is classically defined as "acute" when it occurs within 100 days of transplantation and chronic when it occurs thereafter; however, such a precise distinction from either a clinical or a histopathologic perspective is not justifiable since there is a tremendous overlap [4]. The differential diagnosis of GVHD typically includes both infectious etiologies and reactions to medications (e.g., erythema multiforme), and because neither of these possibilities would respond well to GVHD therapies (i.e., increasing immunosuppressive regimens), the distinction of GVHD from these other dermatologic disorders is clinically very important [4]. An additional important differential diagnostic consideration

M. T. Tetzlaff (✉) · J. L. Curry · V. G. Prieto
Department of Pathology, Section of Dermatopathology, The University of Texas: MD Anderson Cancer Center, 1515 Holcombe Blvd., Unit 85, Houston, TX 77030, USA
e-mail: MTetzlaff@mdanderson.org

© Springer Science+Business Media New York 2015
V. G. Prieto (ed.), *Precision Molecular Pathology of Dermatologic Diseases,*
Molecular Pathology Library 9, DOI 10.1007/978-1-4939-2861-3_7

includes the eruption of lymphocyte recovery [5, 6] and the so-called "engraftment syndrome" [7]. Eruption of lymphocyte recovery is a skin-limited illness with fever which occurs in the first 1–2 weeks following transplantation. It is postulated to be the result of increased skin-specific T cells in the immediate post-engraftment phase and typically resolves with no intervention whatsoever [6]. In contrast, engraftment syndrome is a constellation of fever, erythematous skin rash, and noncardiogenic pulmonary edema that occurs in the immediate phase (1–2 weeks) following both autologous and allogenic transplantation. Engraftment syndrome is due to a complex and intense production of pro-inflammatory cytokines which is considered to be due to general activation of the reconstituted immune system [7]. In addition to histopathologic assessment of skin, liver, and/or gastrointestinal biopsy specimens, molecular approaches including polymerase chain reaction (PCR, see below) and fluorescence in situ hybridization (FISH) techniques have emerged as useful ancillary techniques in the diagnosis of GVHD, particularly in cases where the clinicopathologic presentation is atypical.

This chapter will examine the application of molecular pathology to the problem of specimen misidentification in cutaneous pathology, although the principles already discussed are applicable to specimen identity verification in any organ system. Furthermore, we will explore the application of molecular pathology to the identification of chimerism in patients following stem cell transplantation. In the latter instance, molecular identity testing approaches are critical ancillary techniques to determine the identity of inflammatory cells producing clinical symptoms to direct appropriate management decisions in this relatively rare, but fragile patient population.

Identity Testing: Short Tandem Repeat Polymerase Chain Reaction (STR-PCR)

The human genome contains many different tandemly repeated noncoding DNA sequences [8]. These are typically classified according to the length of the tandemly repeated DNA sequence. *Satellites* contain several thousand base pair (bp) elements of tandemly repeated noncoding DNA. *Minisatellites* are comprised much shorter tandemly repeated noncoding DNA elements of approximately 10–200 bp and are typically 1–5 kilobase pairs (kB) in length overall. Minisatellites are also referred to as *variable number of tandem repeats* (VNTR). Finally, *microsatellites* (also referred to as *short tandem repeats,* STRs) contain ~ 2–7 bp sequences that are tandemly repeated between ~ 5–50 times and generally range in length from ~ 100–300 bp overall [9] .

Because of their small size and relative high degree of polymorphism in the general population, STRs have emerged as powerful tools in human identity testing, including for forensic and paternity identification purposes [8, 10, 11]. In short, polymerase chain reaction (PCR) amplification uses primers flanking a given STR

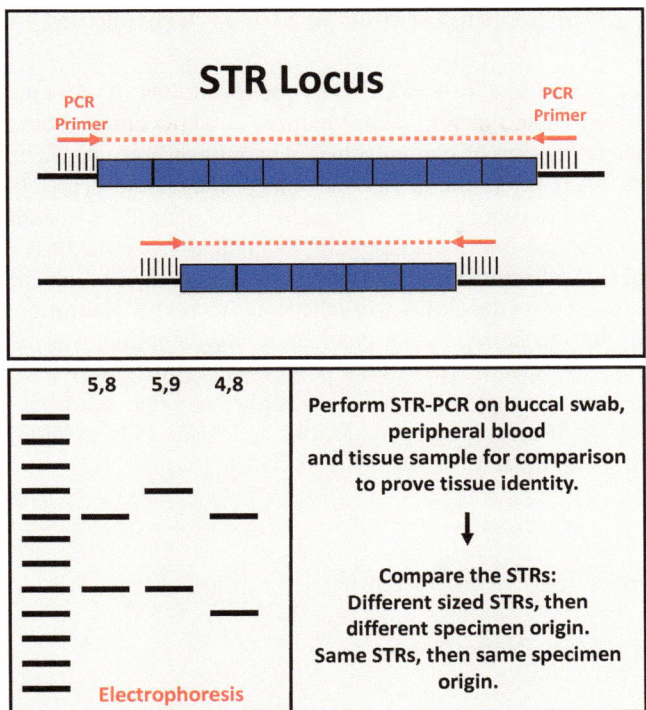

Fig. 7.1 Short tandem repeat (*STR*) testing strategy. (*Top*) Polymerase chain reaction (*PCR*) amplification employs primers flanking a given STR region to amplify that STR. Each STR locus contains a variable number of tandem repeats that are amplified. (*Bottom*) These differences are determined by electrophoresis, which separates the PCR products according to their size

sequence to amplify that STR (Fig. 7.1). As there is variability in the number of repeats among the various alleles for a given STR locus, there is a range of potential sizes of the subsequent PCR products. These differences are determined by electrophoresis, which separates the PCR products according to their size (Fig. 7.1).

Commercially available kits are now readily available that enable the simultaneous amplification of multiple STR loci in a single tube by multiplex PCR [12]. Multiplexing of these STR-PCRs is facilitated by the use of primers labeled with differing fluorescent dyes in combination with a design of distinctly sized STR products. Following STR-PCR, then, the products are size-separated using some form of electrophoresis. Commercially available kits also contain "allelic ladders" which contain all of the known sizes of the most frequently encountered alleles described for a given STR locus. These allelic ladders are subjected to simultaneous electrophoresis, and comparison of the STR-PCR products from a given sample to the allelic ladder defines the relative size/allele of the different STRs interrogated in that sample [8, 10, 11, 13].

Identity Testing: Fluorescence In Situ Hybridization

FISH utilizes fluorescently labeled DNA probes to identify chromosomal alterations in cells. FISH can identify abnormalities of whole chromosomal numbers as well as discrete regions of chromosomes which have been amplified, deleted, or translocated. FISH offers the distinct advantage that fluorescently labeled probes can be hybridized to routine (5 μm) formalin-fixed, paraffin-embedded tissue sections. The number of fluorescent signals per nucleus (described as "dots") can be counted and the cells containing these signals can be morphologically identified. FISH, therefore, offers the ability to evaluate copy number aberrations at a cellular level and further, to correlate any changes in copy number at a particular locus (corresponding to a specific fluorescent probe) with cellular morphology under conventional light microscopy. FISH has been applied to many questions in pathology, including the diagnosis of pigmented lesions in the skin [14], cytology [15], hematologic disorders [16], and the diagnosis of GVHD [17].

Identity Testing: Case Presentation

Is This My Skin Biopsy?

To demonstrate the application of STR-PCR in our clinical practice, we describe the case of a 46-year-old Caucasian woman. She was presented to MD Anderson in 2005, with an approximate 2-year history of a lesion on her right lateral thigh. The patient states that her history began two years earlier when she discovered an erythematous, raised lesion that was symmetrical. Initially, an attempt was made to remove this area with cryotherapy. However, the lesion persisted and then developed a small central area of pigmentation within the last couple of months. Subsequently, she had the lesion removed by a shave biopsy and final pathology revealed invasive melanoma, superficial spreading type, Clark level IV, Breslow thickness of at least 0.6 mm with vertical growth phase (Fig. 7.2).

However, given the clinical history of a predominantly amelanotic lesion that was not originally felt to be clinically suspicious for melanoma, the patient questioned whether the diagnostic skin biopsy, in fact, belonged to her and suggested that specimen misidentification might explain the apparent clinical-pathologic incongruity. She therefore requested DNA identity testing to confirm that the skin biopsy specimen indeed belonged to her. She submitted peripheral blood and buccal swab samples for comparative STR-PCR analysis to the skin biopsy. The STR microsatellite polymorphism pattern of the microdissected tissue from the shave biopsy is identical to the pattern seen from both the peripheral blood and buccal swab samples for all of the eight polymorphic loci examined (Fig. 7.3).

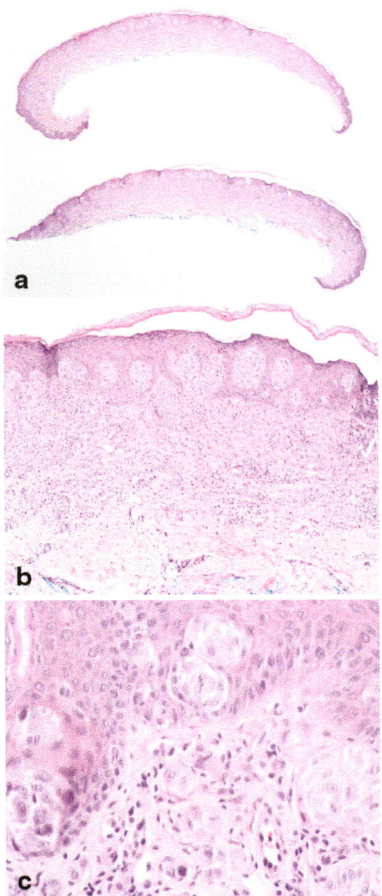

Fig. 7.2 Invasive melanoma on the thigh of a 46-year-old woman. **a** Scanning magnification of shave biopsy specimen demonstrating invasive melanoma with proliferation atypical melanocytes in the epidermis and dermis (4×). **b** Epidermal component with atypical melanocytes disposed as nests and as single cells with pagetoid upward migration. Dermis with invasive melanoma cells with absence of maturation with progressive descent into the reticular dermis (20×). **c** High magnification reveals atypical intraepidermal mitotic figure and atypical dermal melanocytes which lack maturation

Whose Lymphocytes Are They?

We previously described a case of GVHD with an atypical clinical presentation to highlight the utility of molecular diagnostic techniques as a useful ancillary technique in the diagnosis of GVHD [18]. A 25-year-old woman with a history of T cell acute lymphoblastic leukemia (T-ALL) and subsequent acute myelogenous leukemia (AML) underwent umbilical cord hematopoietic stem cell transplantation

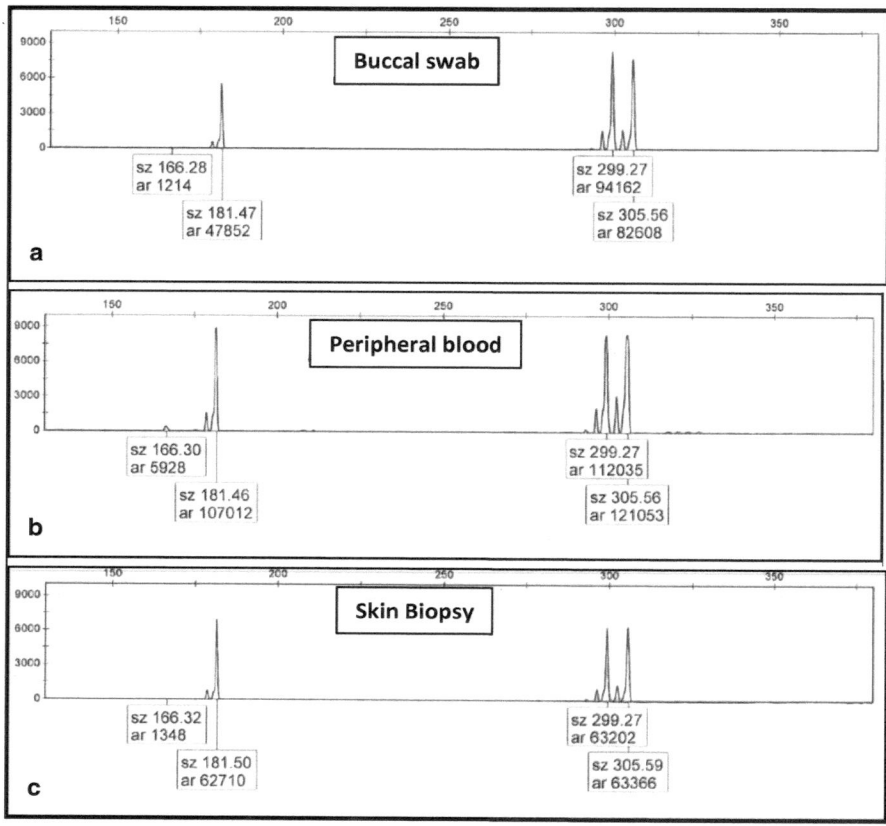

Fig. 7.3 Short tandem repeat (*STR*) testing results for disputed biopsy specimen. Polymerase chain reaction (*PCR*) amplification reveals STR size predominantly 181 at one STR locus and 299 and 305 at a STR different locus on buccal swab tissue (**a**), peripheral blood (**b**) and skin biopsy specimen (**c**). Each STR locus tested showed identical STR fragment length polymorphisms for each of the tissues tested, confirming the identity of the skin biopsy specimen as the patient belonging to the buccal swab and peripheral blood

matched at 4/6 human leukocyte antigen (HLA) loci from a male donor. Eight days following her transplantation, she developed a rash on her ears, face, chest, and arms with an elevated total bilirubin (3.1 U/L; normal range: 0.1–0.5 U/L) and reduced hemoglobin (8.9 g/dL; normal range: 12–16 g/dL), and low white blood cell count (0.6/μL; normal range: 4×10^3–11×10^3/μL). A skin biopsy from an affected area of the chest revealed a paucicellular interface dermatitis characterized by occasional lymphocytes approximating the dermal–epidermal junction with associated vacuolar degeneration of the basal keratinocytes, dyskeratosis, and pigment incontinence. Together with the timing of the onset of clinical symptoms (eight days following stem cell transplantation), these findings were consistent with hyperacute GVHD; however, the differential diagnosis included engraftment syndrome.

Because the stem cell transplant was derived from a male donor, we performed FISH using fluorescently labeled probes corresponding to both the X- and Y-chromosomes to determine whether the lymphocytes at the dermal–epidermal junction were indeed derived from the donor. As shown in Fig. 7.4, FISH highlights many cells containing two X-chromosome signals (red dots) along with a small subset of cells containing XY signals (red and green dots), and these latter cells correspond to the lymphocytes approximating the dermal–epidermal junction.

Together with the clinical and histopathologic findings, these data supported the diagnosis of hyperacute GVHD. Treatment with prednisone (2 mg/kg/d) resulted in improvement of her rash and a decrease in her total bilirubin.

Fig. 7.4 FISH facilitates the diagnosis of GVHD. **a** Skin biopsy of erythematous maculopapular rash on the chest with basket weave stratum corneum and hypocellular interface dermatitis with necrotic keratinocytes (10×). **b** FISH analysis with cells containing two X-chromosome signals (*red dots*) mixed with a subset of cells containing XY signals (*red* and *green dots*) with nuclei indicated by a 4′,6-diamidino-2-phenylindole (*DAPI*) fluorescent counterstain. The latter cells are interpreted as the lymphocytes approximating the dermal–epidermal junction (20×). Dotted line indicates the approximate dermal–epidermal junction

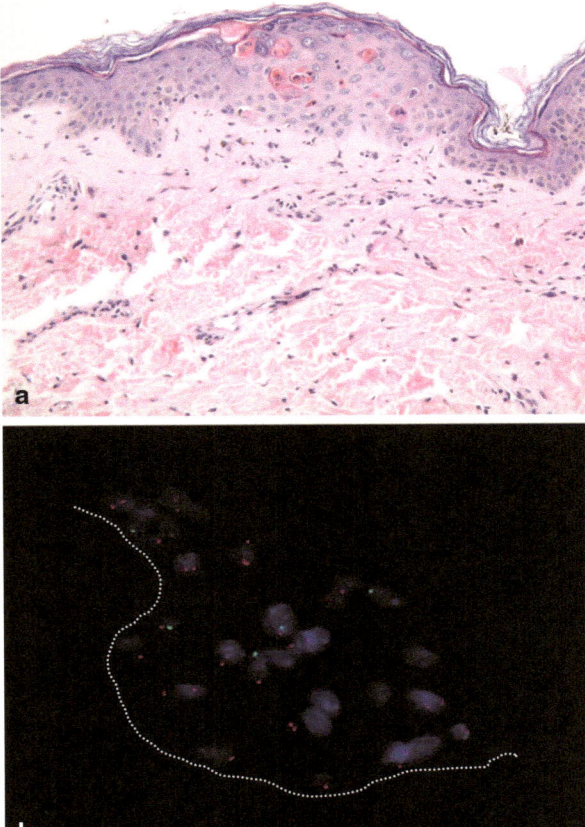

Conclusion

Similar to other disciplines in surgical pathology, the field of cutaneous pathology has enlisted many molecular approaches to facilitate tissue identification and cellular identification at the molecular level. These molecular tools have had profound clinical applications in diagnosis, management decisions, and outcomes. Additional information on the molecular tests available at the Molecular Diagnostic Laboratory at the University of Texas MD Anderson Cancer Center, Houston, Texas can be found at the website: (http://www.mdanderson.org/education-and-research/resources-for-professionals/scientific-resources/core-facilities-and-services/molecular-diagnostics-lab/index.html)

References

1. Layfield LJ, Anderson GM. Specimen labeling errors in surgical pathology: an 18-month experience. Am J Clin Pathol. 2010;134(3):466.
2. Marberger M, McConnell JD, Fowler I, et al. Biopsy misidentification identified by DNA profiling in a large multicenter trial. J Clin Oncol. 2011;29(13):1744.
3. Troxel DB. Error in surgical pathology. Am J Surg Pathol. 2004;28(8):1092.
4. Deeg HJ, Antin JH. The clinical spectrum of acute graft-versus-host disease. Semin Hematol. 2006;43(1):24.
5. Bauer DJ, Hood AF, Horn TD. Histologic comparison of autologous graft-vs-host reaction and cutaneous eruption of lymphocyte recovery. Arch Dermatol. 1993;129(7):855.
6. Horn TD, Redd JV, Karp JE, Beschorner WE, Burke PJ, Hood AF. Cutaneous eruptions of lymphocyte recovery. Arch Dermatol. 1989;125(11):1512.
7. Spitzer TR. Engraftment syndrome following hematopoietic stem cell transplantation. Bone Marrow Transplant. 2001;27(9):893.
8. Hohoff C, Brinkmann B. Human identity testing with PCR-based systems. Mol Biotechnol. 1999;13(2):123.
9. Edwards A, Civitello A, Hammond HA, Caskey CT. DNA typing and genetic mapping with trimeric and tetrameric tandem repeats. Am J Hum Genet. 1991;49(4):746.
10. Butler JM. Genetics and genomics of core short tandem repeat loci used in human identity testing. J Forensic Sci. 2006;51(2):253.
11. Butler JM. Short tandem repeat typing technologies used in human identity testing. Biotechniques. 2007;43(4):ii.
12. Wang DY, Chang CW, Lagace RE, Calandro LM, Hennessy LK. Developmental Validation of the AmpFlSTR((R)) Identifiler((R)) Plus PCR Amplification Kit: An Established Multiplex Assay with Improved Performance. J Forensic Sci. 2011;56(4):835–45.
13. Tracey M. Short tandem repeat-based identification of individuals and parents. Croat Med J. 2001;42(3):233.
14. Gerami P, Zembowicz A. Update on fluorescence in situ hybridization in melanoma: state of the art. Arch Pathol Lab Med. 2011;135(7):830.
15. Bubendorf L, Grilli B, Sauter G, Mihatsch MJ, Gasser TC, Dalquen P. Multiprobe FISH for enhanced detection of bladder cancer in voided urine specimens and bladder washings. Am J Clin Pathol. 2001;116(1):79.
16. Sreekantaiah C. FISH panels for hematologic malignancies. Cytogenet Genome Res. 2007;118(2–4):284.

17. Au WY, Ma SK, Kwong YL, et al. Graft-versus-host disease after liver transplantation: documentation by fluorescent in situ hybridisation and human leucocyte antigen typing. Clin Transplant. 2000;14(2):174.
18. Nguyen J, Tetzlaff MT, Zhang PJ, Xu X, Hexner E, Rosenbach M. Fluorescent in situ hybridization of a skin biopsy: an adjunctive tool to support a diagnosis of graft-versus-host disease. J Am Acad Dermatol. 2011;64(6):e113.

Index

© Springer Science+Business Media New York 2015
V. G. Prieto (ed.), *Precision Molecular Pathology of Dermatologic Diseases,*
Molecular Pathology Library 9, DOI 10.1007/978-1-4939-2861-3